This is not your normal weight loss ~~~~~~~~~~~~~~~~~~~~~~~~~~ gets to the core issue of weight for many of us—our spiritual health. Penny combines her years of professional experience and her personal journey of faith to inspire and encourage us to face those thoughts that bind us to our struggle with weight.
—*Kristin Miller, M.S., R.D., L.D., Clinical Dietitian*

This book integrates biblical and nutritional expertise. Penny has a step-by-step way to lose weight with God's help. It's easy to read with an enriching daily devotion. It's a testimony of putting God in control of every part of your life including your weight. Start living healthier with Christ in control!
—*Vivian McGarrity, R.D., L.D., Community Dietitian*

Penny has given us a truly wonderful approach to weight loss. With this plan you can lose weight and keep it off. After all, with God's help, how can we fail?
—*Michael B. Shrock, DO, Board certified by American Board of Family Medicine: member American Academy of Family Practice, Mississippi State Medical Association, Mississippi Osteopathic Medical Association*

We make choices every day. Some good, some bad. The way we choose our foods has a major impact on our health and well being. This book helps us understand the food choices we make and the way it affects our life.
—*Jan Todd RN MSN, Family Nurse Practitioner*

Living a healthy lifestyle and managing your weight in today's culture is extremely difficult for the average person. Penny not only puts forth a common sense plan, but also a biblically based one, continually reminding the believer that we have One on our side who enables us to do all things!
—*Rev. Tod Thompson*

The 40-DAY Diet Makeover

A Daily Journey with God to a New You!

Penny W. Dickerson, M.S., R.D., L.D.

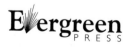

Evergreen PRESS

Mobile, Alabama

ISBN 978-1-58169-358-4
For Worldwide Distribution
Printed in the U.S.A.

Evergreen Press
P.O. Box 191540 • Mobile, AL 36619
800-367-8203

Table of Contents

Acknowledgments

I praise God for allowing me to be used by Him to write this program. May God receive the glory for every good and perfect thing reaped from this book.

God has blessed me by surrounding me with a team of Christian dietitians who have been very instrumental in the completion of this project. A very warm and heartfelt thanks go to Kristin Miller, Shannon Kuntz, and Vivian McGarrity. Their advice, contributions, expertise, and editing skills have been a very valuable asset to this study. Their friendship, patience, and endless support have also been such a blessing. They are truly gifts from God. I could not have done this without them.

God has also blessed me by bringing people into my life who have been willing to come with me and be godly friends and mentors. Art Starkey, who very graciously agreed to edit this study, your expertise and willingness to give of your time and energy to a project so dear to my heart means the world to me. God bless you and Connie for her proofreading skills.

Rev. George McFarland, thank you for sharing your expertise so graciously.

I would also like to thank the love of my life, my husband, Kenny, for believing in me. Thanks also to my three sons, Spencer, Taylor, and Hunter for your love and patience. Having such unwavering support from the guys in my life has meant more to me than you will ever know. I am truly blessed with a godly husband, godly parents, and a family I know I can always depend on to lift me up with praises and prayers.

Then I heard the voice of the Lord saying, "Whom shall I send? And who will go for us?" And I said, "Here am I. Send Me!" (Isaiah 6:8).

To God be the glory!

This book is dedicated to my biggest fans:

my loving husband, Kenny

my sons, Spencer, Taylor, and Hunter

and my parents, Max and Virginia West

for all your love

and unwavering support

Disclaimer

The exercises and dietary suggestions in this book are intended for healthy individuals. If you have medical problems, a physical disability, or are unsure whether or not you should do certain exercises, please consult a medical professional.

The Beginning of Your Journey

So whether you eat or drink or whatever you do, do it all for the glory of God (1 Corinthians 10:31).

Your journey to a lifetime of weight management and healthy living begins today with *The 40-Day Diet Makeover.* As you know, most diets only work when you stay on them, then as soon as you get off them the results quickly dissipate. Often the on again/off again journey results in some—or all—of the weight being regained. *The 40-Day Diet Makeover* will provide you with the tools you need to makeover your diet by changing your eating habits to help you achieve permanent weight loss. Therefore, it is a lifestyle to be developed, not a diet to remain on.

This program will take you through the process of making changes in what you eat and how you live, which will result in a lifetime of weight management and wellness. This guide will explore the spiritual, physical, and emotional issues associated with healthy living.

The 40-Day Diet Makeover is a biblically based weight loss program designed for success. Unlike fad diets, which rely on certain foods or gimmicks to help you lose weight, this program is designed to help you develop a partnership with God so He can help you use the foods He has given you to glorify Him.

In fact, the focus of this program is to honor God with your body. Have you ever thought about asking God for help with your diet? God wants to be a part of every aspect of your life including your struggle with your weight. Luke 11:9-10 says,

So I say to you: Ask and it will be given to you; seek and you will find; knock and the door will be opened to you. For everyone who asks receives; he who seeks finds; and to him who knocks, the door will be opened.

Sometimes your prayers may simply need to be one word, "Help!" God will not intervene in your life and help you unless you ask Him. He needs an invitation from you. Until you humble yourself and ask Him for help,

1

He will not help. During your 40-day journey to a better weight, you will learn to invoke God's help and apply basic principles of nutrition to develop a healthy lifestyle that will last a lifetime.

How To Make Your Journey Work for You

As you work through this program, you will find that each day builds on the previous one. Take time to study the information and work through the daily devotions as you spend time in God's Word. Implement the suggested changes into your diet and lifestyle daily. Those changes, the devotions, and the knowledge you glean from each day will work together to lead you to a lifetime of weight management. Each day the devotion will also give you various kinds of information, tips, and challenges. There is also a space for daily prayer journaling and for food journaling in a food diary. Prayer journaling is a very powerful way to invite God to be a part of your day-to-day struggles and to employ His help on your journey.

Keeping a food diary is essential to maintaining a lifetime of weight management and wellness. Studies show that food journaling is one of the best predictors of success in any weight management program. Start today documenting each bite of food, candy, or gum and each beverage you drink from the time you get up until the time you go to bed. Some people have no idea how much food they are eating in a day. By writing it down, you will be able to see how much you are really consuming, discover your typical times of overeating, and identify any problem behaviors. You may need to take a notepad with you to work or keep it in your vehicle so you will not miss cataloguing any of the food you eat.

Keeping track of your weight is also a very important part of this program. After all, how can you know when you are making progress if you don't keep track of your weight from the beginning? If you don't have a scale, I strongly suggest you invest in one or borrow one from a friend. During the program, you will be asked to chart your weight progress once a week on the weight tracking grid provided.

Start at zero, then each following week put an "X" in the box corresponding with your weight decrease, increase, or maintenance. For example, if during Week 2 you lost two pounds, then you would put an "X" in the "–2" box in the Week 2 column.

Weight Tracking Grid

Starting Weight: _299.2_   Starting Date: March 28th 2016

Week	1	2	3	4	5	6	7	8	9	10	11	12	13	14	15
+ 9															
+ 8															
+ 7															
+ 6															
+ 5															
+ 4															
+ 3															
+ 2															
+ 1															
0	X														
- 1															
- 2															
- 3															
- 4															
- 5															
- 6															
- 7															
- 8															
- 9															
- 10															
- 11															
- 12															
- 13															
- 14															
- 15															
- 16															
- 17															
- 18															
- 19															
- 20															
- 21															
- 22															
- 23															
- 24															
- 25															
- 26															
- 27															
- 28															
- 29															
- 30															
Week	1	2	3	4	5	6	7	8	9	10	11	12	13	14	15

Begin here ●◆ (at row 0)

3

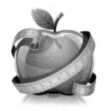

Day 1

Who Is in Control—You or the Food?

Commit to the Lord whatever you do, and your plans will succeed (Proverbs 16:3).

Commitment. This simple word carries so much significance for the success of this program. Are you truly ready to commit? Are you ready to make the changes and sacrifices in your lifestyle necessary to help you lose weight? The *40-Day Diet Makeover* is not magic; it requires true commitment, big sacrifices, and a lot of hard work. The good news is, you are not alone; you have a partner, God, who will provide the extra self-control and strength you need to help you stay on your journey.

The *40-Day Diet Makeover* will give you pertinent information about nutrition to help you make informed decisions about healthy food choices. It is also designed to help you discover the power of God and His Word in helping you with weight management and developing a healthy lifestyle. Through this program you will develop beneficial, lasting habits that will enhance your daily living.

Work through the daily devotion as you began your journey. Use the devotion with your Bible and set aside some time each day to daily meditate on God's Word. There will be Scriptures for you to look up throughout the program. As you work through the book, dedicate yourself to making gradual, cumulative, and lasting changes in your lifestyle and eating habits, which will help you reap the lasting results of weight loss.

As you begin your journey through *The 40-Day Diet Makeover*, also be prepared to:

- Increase your physical activity.
- Cook healthier.
- Learn to make wise and healthy food choices.
- Pay closer attention to what and how much you eat.
- Get in tune with your body's God given ability to lose weight and keep it off.

The first step of this program is to determine your state of readiness. Take a moment to fill out the Readiness Questionnaire below. When you have completed the questionnaire, move on to the Day One Daily Devotion.

Readiness Questionnaire

1. Have you ever been on a diet?

Yes Many times

2. Why did you get off it?

lazy NO commitment, want to eat whatever NO will power

3. Think about something to which you are truly devoted. Maybe it is a job, going to school, a marriage, raising children, a church, or a community activity. List all the factors that keep you committed.

a. *love*
b. *good lifestyle*
c. *happiness*
d.
e.

4. Can you find that same kind of persevering spirit to dedicate to this program? This program will require serious diligence to be successful. Are you ready to wholeheartedly commit to making the sacrifices it will take to develop a healthy lifestyle?

"Commit to the Lord whatever you do and your plans will succeed" (Proverbs 16:3). Before you begin your journey through *The 40-Day Diet Makeover*, spend some time on your knees in prayer. Ask God to help you get to a state of readiness. Dedicate this program to Him and ask for His help.

Daily Devotion — Day 1

Read Ephesians 3:15-20. Key verse: Ephesians 3:16, which says:

> *I pray that out of His glorious riches He may strengthen you with power through His Spirit in your inner being.*

Now apply this word to yourself: I pray that out of His glorious riches He may strengthen __Kay__ (your name) with power through His Spirit in my inner being.

Physical Challenges for Today

The USDA Dietary Guidelines, which we will cover later, can be very helpful when incorporated into your eating habits. They include some simple steps towards a healthier lifestyle. The basic recommendations are:

- Increase fruit.
- Increase colored vegetables.
- Increase low fat dairy.
- Increase whole grain foods.
- Increase lean meats.
- Decrease fats, salt, and sugar.

Your nutrition challenge:
Pick one guideline or recommendation on which to focus each week.

Your fitness challenge:
Increase the intensity of your physical activity this week.

God will supply you with the courage to change!

🍎 **Food Diary**	🙏 **Your Prayer**
B: water apple 2 WW toast Pnut Butter.	Heavenly Father, Thank you for everything I have been blessed with, My kids, My husband our home and jobs. Please give me strength to be healthier- So I can lose weight Please Help Me stick to it so I can lose the weight and help my family be healthier. Please show me where I can be helpful to you. I love you. Amen.

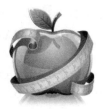

Day 2

God Helps Us With Our Struggles

How does God fit into your life? Do you call on Him the moment your eyes open in the morning? Do you praise Him for your life and for bringing you to this point?

God has a perfect plan for you. He wants to use every struggle and every trial you face for His glory. The only way He can do this is through your praise of Him, your acceptance of your current circumstances, and your trust in Him for the future. Every problem and struggle you've experienced have brought you to this point in your life. God loves you and will use your struggles to prepare you for a time such as this.

Praise God for the life He has given you and for all the events that have happened to bring you to this point. Then praise Him for the work He is about to do in your life through your journey to lose weight. God inhabits our praises. When we accept our current situation and praise God for it, He can use it for His glory.

Take a moment to tell God you realize that you are overweight and struggle with food. Thank Him for your life just as it is. Praise Him for every obstacle you have faced and will face in the future, and ask Him to use those obstacles for His glory. Thank God because He loves you no matter what. Ask Him to carry you through your journey and on to victory.

Calculating Your Body Mass Index

Calculate your Body Mass Index (BMI). BMI is an important indicator that medical professionals use to diagnose your risk for developing heart disease, diabetes, hypertension, and certain cancers. It is a good ruler to gauge body weight and body fat ratios. BMI values apply to men and women regardless of age, muscle mass, or frame size. Use this calculation with other health indicators as a guide on your wellness journey. Calculate your BMI using the following formula:

Step 1 _____ ÷ _____ = _____
           (Weight)   (Height in inches)   (A)

Step 2 _____ ÷ _____ = _____
          (Answer A)   (Height in inches)   (B)

Step 3 _____ x   704.5   = _____
          (Answer B)   BMI

A BMI of less than 18 is considered underweight.

A BMI of 18.5 - 25 is considered healthy.

A BMI of 25 - 30 is considered overweight.

A BMI of 30 is considered obese.

> *Note: These values don't apply to athletes, body builders, pregnant and nursing women, frail or elderly persons, or persons under eighteen.*

The truth about your BMI can be painful, especially if you have always considered yourself just overweight but you find you are really obese. This should help give you an idea of where you are and where you need to be for long-term weight goals. People who are overweight or obese have a greater chance of developing high blood pressure, cholesterol, type 2 diabetes, heart disease, stroke, and certain types of cancers. Realizing the fact your weight may be putting you in serious health risk should help motivate you to persevere.

One point I must stress is the importance of a slow, gradual weight loss of one to two pounds per week. Remember, this is not a diet; it is a lifestyle because you are making over your diet and eating habits to result in gradual, *permanent* weight loss.

One of the reasons fad diets don't work is they promote losing large amounts of weight quickly. If you lose weight too quickly from unrealistic changes in your eating habits, which you cannot maintain, you will be doomed to gaining weight back when your eating habits return to normal. If you are making lasting lifestyle changes, the result will be gradual weight loss that will last a lifetime.

Of course we are all different sizes. God did not make us all look alike, and we don't all fit into the same box. You may never be as little as you think you would like to be, but you can be healthy at any size. Therefore, keep the following points in mind:

- Set realistic weight goals so you don't set yourself up for failure.
- Think about the lowest you have weighed in the past five to ten years: _____ pounds. Perhaps you may want to start with that weight as an initial goal.
- You may not be able to lose all the weight you would like to lose, but statistics show that even a 10 percent reduction in weight will help decrease your health risk greatly. What is 10 percent of your current weight? _____ pounds. This amount would be another option for your initial weight loss goal.

God loves you more than you can ever imagine. Cherish that love; don't wait until you reach a certain weight loss to start feeling good about yourself. Do your best to be healthy whatever your weight is. Start today praising God for your life and praising Him for helping you be successful in getting the weight off. Let His love flow from you. Find your contentment in Him so you can find true happiness at every stage of your journey.

Pause now for a moment in God's Word.

Daily Devotion — Day 2

Read Matthew 26:36-45. Key verse: Matthew 26:41. Fill in the blanks.

"Watch and _____ so that you will not fall into _____.
The _____ is willing but the _____ is weak."

Physical Challenges for Today ✔

Let's review and fill in the blanks below.

1. What kind of issues do you struggle with when it comes to food? Overeating? Craving sweets? Do you love fried foods?

_____

_____

2. Your daily journey to weight management is not a diet it is a

_____.

3. A realistic weight loss goal is _____ pounds each week.

4. What is your BMI goal? _____

Ask God to give you supernatural self-control today!

Your nutrition challenge:
Decrease your portion sizes
from what you currently serve yourself.

Your fitness challenge:
Walk one-half mile today.

🍎 Food Diary	🙏 Your Prayer

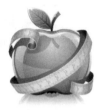

DAY 3

Battle of the Bulge

In this program we will be exploring ways to let God fight every battle we face, even the battle of the bulge. Remember that *The 40-Day Diet Makeover* is not a diet; it is a lifestyle. It will help you renovate your diet and eating habits for a lifetime. You need to be open to making permanent changes in your eating habits for this program to be successful. Most health problems don't start with a single event in your life; rather, they are from an accumulation of events over the years. Therefore, those problems can't be corrected with a single diet or pill.

Lists, sticky notes, and day planners are an essential part of my life. Without them I would never remember all the items I must shop for at the grocery store, the need to pick up my husband's shirts from the laundry, or the meeting I have to attend at two o'clock this afternoon. Lists make me more organized, help me stay on task, and aid me in remembering my commitments. How about you? What keeps you on track? What is going to keep you committed in your journey to lose weight?

You can start with a commitment to food journaling. Food journaling is keeping a list of the exact amounts of all the food you eat in a day. This can be done on a neat and organized food diary like the special one in this chapter, which is divided up into various meals, or it can be done on a notebook you set up just for that purpose, or as a part of each day's devotion in the space provided at the end of each Day's Journey. If your memory is not very good, you may want to keep a little pocket-sized notebook in your purse or pocket so you can keep up with it as you are eating. The way you choose to keep the food diary is not important; the fact that you do it faithfully is.

Food journaling is one of the best predictors of success in any weight management program. The concept is if you write it down, you are going to pay closer attention to what you are eating and therefore eat less. As a general rule, most people pay very little attention to the food they are putting in their mouths.

Food journaling helps you see where most of your fat and calories are coming from and helps you identify those areas in which you need to improve. Of course, this tool will not work if you are not honest. For the most benefit, you need to record every single item you put in your mouth (estimating the amount is fine).

If kept faithfully, food journaling can be one of the most helpful tools you have. It is useful for identifying emotional triggers or times during the day when you may need to improve your eating habits.

Start your food journal or diary today. It may be helpful to find a partner with whom you can share your food diaries, someone who will hold you accountable and help keep you motivated.

Did You Know?

Prayer journaling, like food journaling, is one of the most helpful tools you have. It makes your prayers more powerful! As you look back at your prayers, the journal helps you remember what you prayed and see how often your prayers are being answered. This reminds you to praise God for answered prayers. Take advantage of the daily food and prayer journals after each devotion.

Daily Devotion — Day 3

Read 1 Thessalonians 5:12-22. Key verses: 1 Thessalonians 5:16-18.

Fill in the blanks.

Be joyful _____ ; pray _____ ; give thanks in all circumstances, for this is God's will for you in Christ Jesus.

Most of us live our lives in the pursuit of happiness, thinking happiness is the source of our joy. In reality, happiness is an emotion dependent on personal feelings.

Joy is the unconditional state of mind that accompanies fellowship with God. It is characterized by great well-being. Joy is a Spirit-given gift that flourishes best in hard times.

The problem with happiness is its lack of permanence. It can be cancelled without further notice due to an accident, loss of a loved one, a divorce, or any unexpected tragedy that rocks your world and turns it upside down. On the other hand, godly joy carries a lifetime warranty. Not derived from or dependent on conditions, circumstances cannot take joy away. The joy of the Lord brings strength (Nehemiah 8:10). Joy is a motivating factor that propels us over the rough terrain we often have to travel.

If you find pressures of circumstances disrupt your relationship with God and take away your good feelings, then maybe you are relying upon happiness rather than true joy. If those same pressures do not disrupt your joy but drive you toward God, then you know you have found real joy.

Joy is the echo of God's life within us!

Food Diary	Your Prayer

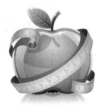

Day 4

Become Like a Child

Let's start from the beginning. From the time you were born, did you realize God has given you many instincts to help you control your weight?

Look up Genesis 2:7 in your Bible and fill in the blanks.

The Lord God _____ the man from the _____ of the ground and breathed into his nostrils the _____ of life, and the man became a _____ being.

When God formed man, He built in many instincts and mechanisms to help with weight management. Let's start by looking at a baby. With what eating instincts are babies born?

Have you ever held a newborn and noticed every time you touched his or her check, the baby turns toward you and open his or her mouth, especially if the infant is breastfeeding? This is called a rooting reflex; it is a baby's God-given instinct to look for food.

Have you ever seen kittens right after they are born? They have the same rooting reflex; they will nudge around on their mother until they find a nipple to nurse while their eyes are not even open. If babies were not given the instinct to suck, they would starve to death. Babies also stop eating when they are full and spit up when they've had too much.

God made our stomachs so we hold only a certain amount of food at a time. The problem is, unlike a baby, we don't spit up when we have had too much. The more we stuff ourselves, the bigger our stomachs get. The more food our stomachs will hold, the more fat we store and the more pounds we pack on to our bodies.

Children also have many built-in instincts to help them control their weight. I have three boys. It has been interesting to watch the different stages of their development as they have grown. Have you ever tried to get a child to eat who is not hungry? It is almost impossible, isn't it? When my boys were younger, I used to prepare a nice big meal for them only to have their father and me be the only ones to eat all of it. One of the three might eat well one night and another eat well the next night.

If children are following their instincts, they will only eat when they are hungry. If they are experiencing a growth spurt, they will eat like crazy. At other times, they may just push their food around on their plate and only eat a few bites of their favorite food.

People always told me when my boys were little that one day they would eat. I have made it to the teenage years with two of the boys, and now they sure do eat! Teenage boys can put away a ton of food—2,500-4,000 calories/day—especially when they are playing sports. I now keep our local grocery store in business.

The point is, we should all try to be more like our children. They are more in tune with their bodies; they generally eat when they are hungry and stop eating when they are full. The rise in childhood obesity in America is mainly due to inactivity and parents' poor eating habits spilling over to younger children.

Look up Matthew 18:3 and fill in the blanks.

And [Jesus] said: "I tell you the _____, unless you change and become like little _____, you will never enter the kingdom of _____."

Ask God to help you rebirth those instincts He gave you at birth on your journey to weight management. Ask Him to help you become more in tune with your body. Eat only when you are hungry and learn to stop eating when you feel full. You need to make a conscious effort to be more active as well.

Pause for a moment in God's Word.

Daily Devotion — Day 4

Read Psalm 119:9-16. Key verses: Psalm 119:9-11. Fill in the blanks.

How can a young man keep his way pure? By living according to your _____. I seek you with all my _____; do not let me stray from your _____. I have hidden your word in my heart that I might not sin against you.

```
  0                          5                          10
```

On this scale from 0-10, with 0 meaning you have not accepted Jesus as your Lord and Savior and 10 being perfection (you have placed every aspect of your life in His hands and hold nothing back), how would you rate your current walk with God? Put a mark with a date beside it on the line above representing where you now are.

- Are you walking with Him daily?

- How often do you read your Bible?

You cannot know Christ without knowing His Word. You must get into His Word so you can apply it to your life.

Your spiritual challenge:
Strive to improve your walk with God
so you can be close to the 10 on the scale.

Your fitness challenge:
Increase your activity level today by taking one
30 minute walk or three 10 minute walks today.

🍎 Food Diary	🙏 Your Prayer

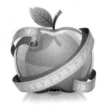

DAY 5

How Long Have You Been
Developing Your Eating Habits?

Did your parents, grandparents, or guardians help you lose some of those instincts with which you were born? Are you helping your children or grandchildren lose them? Were any of the following statements made to you as a child?

"You have to eat everything on your plate before you can leave the table."

"Eat it whether you like it or not."

"You must eat everything on your plate before you can have this delicious dessert."

Do you use these same words to the children in your life in order to get them to eat? Are you a member of the "Clean Plate Club"? If these ideas have been drilled into your head as a child, then it makes it difficult for you not to feel like you always have to clean your plate as an adult. You feel guilty when you leave food on your plate. You think about those poor staving children in another country, and you eat it all so you aren't wasting. After all, waste not—want not. How many times have you heard that?

That kind of "stinking thinking" is what is probably contributing to your weight problem. You need to break the cycle by making a conscious effort to put less food on your plate and allow your children to do the same; then do not make yourself or them clean their plate at every meal. Think about it, would you rather have the extra fat and calories on you in the form of pounds, or would you rather they be fed to the dog or put in the trash? Wouldn't it be worth wasting a little food in the name of losing weight?

Eating just a few more calories than your body needs in the name of "cleaning your plate" can be detrimental to your weight loss goals. For instance, if you eat just three extra bites of macaroni and cheese, or four extra bites of cherry pie, or one extra half piece of cornbread at one meal per day, every day for a year, you could gain up to twenty-five pounds. So you see, it is vital to stop eating when you feel full regardless of how much food is left on your plate.

Were you a chubby as a child? Were your parents always putting you on a diet, restricting foods, or using food for reward or punishment? If so, you were probably more likely to want to hoard or sneak food as a child and even as an adult.

Do you ever reward yourself with food? Do you say to yourself, *If I am good and drink this diet soda, then I can eat this candy bar; or I was really good all week, so I am going to reward myself with an extra large chocolate milkshake.* Food should not be used as a reward. A better way to reward yourself is to start a clothing fund. Every time you feel you deserve a reward, put a token amount of money into the fund to go toward the new wardrobe you will be able to purchase when you have reached your weight goal. Rewarding yourself with food will only sabotage all the hard work you have put into eating healthier.

Take a moment to do some soul searching. Try to identify the eating habits and false thinking that may be contributing to your weight problem. What changes do you need to make today to break that cycle? Identifying the core to your eating problems is one of the first steps in dealing with them.

As you work through your devotion, say a prayer that God will help you deal with the issues you have just identified.

Daily Devotion — Day 5

Read 1 Corinthians 6:12-20. Key verses: 1 Corinthians 6:19-20. Fill in the blanks.

Do you not know that your body is a temple of the
_____, who is in you, whom you have received from
_____? You are not your _____; you were bought at a
price. Therefore _____ _____ with your body.

1. Why do you think you are overweight?

2. What are the habits you have had since childhood that may be contributing to your weight problem?

Pray that God will help you start changing some of those specific habits this week. Learn to be comfortable in your own skin. God created you in His image. Strive for a realistic weight where you can be healthy and happy.

Your spiritual challenge:
On your journey, take it one small change at a time,
starting each day with prayer.

🍎 Food Diary	🙏 Your Prayer

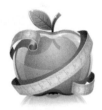

DAY 6

Rebirth Your Instincts

God has given you the ability to tell when you are hungry and when you are full. But if you ignore those sensations long enough, they will go away, which is the case for many of us. Therefore, you need to rebirth those instincts and get back in tune with your body's built-in sensors. Remind yourself on a daily basis that you don't always have to clean your plate.

It takes twenty minutes for your brain to tell your stomach you are full so you need to learn to stop eating before you feel full. You can eat a lot of food in twenty minutes. Stop eating before you feel full even if you have only eaten three-fourths of your plate. Get up and walk around a little or clean up the kitchen, making sure you are still hungry before going back to eat a second helping. If you do go back for seconds, choose more of the vegetables or salad and less of the higher calorie foods.

You need to train yourself to be satisfied with less. Fix your plate like you would normally, then put half of it back. When you are not hungry, don't eat—even if it is mealtime, or the food smells good, or you have had it before and know it is going to taste good. I am not saying to skip meals; you need regular meals at regular intervals. But if you are really not very hungry, your meal can be a light snack—a banana and a cup of yogurt, for example, instead of a big meal. Studies show people who eat two meals a day eat more calories a day than those who eat three meals and a couple of snacks every day.

Let's compare your body to a car. A car needs a constant supply of gas to run properly, just as we need a constant supply of energy to function. Say you go to the gas station and pay for $60 worth of gas. You start pumping only to find that your tank only holds $40 worth of gas, but since you paid for $60, you keep pumping the gas, causing it to spill over the ground. That would be crazy, wouldn't it?

It is also crazy to put more food into your body at one time than your body needs for energy because, unlike a gas tank, your body can hold more than you need. Think about what happens to those extra calories you have eaten. Unfortunately, extra calories equal extra fat and pounds, which will be added to your hips and waistline. On the other hand, if you have no gas, you will have no go! Your body must have a steady supply of calories—our body's fuel—to have energy for everyday activities.

Imagine yourself driving down the road when suddenly you start getting warning signs that you are running out of gas. First, the little red gaslight appears. You say, "Oh, I can go a good twenty miles after this light comes on," so you ignore it. Before you know it, you've already traveled twenty miles further, and you hear a little dinging noise. You are at a critical state now; you must get to the gas station right away or you will be walking. Unfortunately you are out of luck—no gas stations around. You end up stuck on the side of the road, wishing you had not ignored that first warning sign. That is the way your body works.

Let's say you are a person who doesn't eat breakfast. You get up in the morning with just enough time to take a shower, get dressed, get the kids on the bus, and get to work. Who has time to eat in the morning anyway? Your morning seems to be going fine until about ten o'clock, when you start getting hungry. Like your car, your body starts to give you warning signs that you are running on empty.

You get a headache but you are busy, so you take some medicine or some black coffee—for the caffeine of course—and keep going, ignoring the first warning sign. You rock on a couple more hours. By noon, you are running on empty and your body has started giving you every warning sign that it can, attempting to tell you that it is going to be shutting down soon. You get the shakes, you get weak, and you feel as though you are going to pass out if you do not get something to eat.

So what do you do? You go get the biggest, juiciest hamburger you can get, with the super sized fries and a thick, chocolate milkshake. You also end up having a snack in the afternoon and second helpings at supper because you have been starving all day. It is a vicious cycle that will result in your taking in too many calories that spill over to unwanted fat and pounds.

If you had started your day with a healthy breakfast, you could have broken the cycle before it ever started. If you are not a breakfast eater, you might want to consider changing your habits for the sake of your diet.

The word breakfast comes from the concept of "fasting." Fasting is a period of time that you are abstaining from food. When you get up in the morning, ten to twelve hours have passed since you last ate; therefore, it is necessary for you to eat and "break" your "fast." This is why eating breakfast is so important.

Your breakfast does not have to be a big, traditional meal. It could be a granola bar and a glass of milk or juice, a leftover piece of pizza, a peanut butter and jelly sandwich, or a cup of yogurt and a piece of fruit. In fact, it would be better for you to choose something a little lighter for breakfast than the traditional sausage biscuit, loaded with fat and calories. You also don't have to eat this meal as soon as you wake up. You can eat later in the morning. If you work, plan ahead and take something to work with you and eat it after you arrive. Having a healthy breakfast is a great way to start off the day.

If you eat breakfast, you may not be as likely to be as hungry at lunch, which will allow you to choose a healthier lunch: a small hamburger, small French fries, and a diet drink instead of a super sized burger and fries with a milkshake. You can have a smaller, healthier snack in the afternoon: a piece of fruit or a bag of 100 calorie popcorn. Supper could consist of smaller servings.

If you spread out your calories throughout the day, controlling the amount of food you eat will be easier. Spreading your food into small amounts throughout the day allows your body to have energy as your body needs it—in small amounts. That will help you control your weight.

Not eating or skipping meals in the name of "dieting" is going to lead to dieting disaster. Try it for a few weeks. Monitor yourself on a day you are eating two meals versus a day you eat three meals and two to three snacks, and see which day you take in more calories. Use your food diary to help you monitor your intake. I bet you will find you do better eating small amounts more frequently. It will also help you feel as though you are not even on a diet because you will be eating all the time.

Pause now for a moment in God's Word.

Daily Devotion — Day 6

Read Galatians 5:13-17. Key verses: Galatians 5:16-17.

Fill in the blanks:

So I say, live by the _____ and you will not _____ the
desires of the _____ _____. For the _____
_____ desires what is contrary to the _____, and the
_____ what is contrary to the sinful nature. They are in
_____ with each other, so that you do not do what you want.

God will prompt you to do what you need to do to help you move
toward a healthier diet and lifestyle if you ask Him to. However,
you will probably have to battle with your flesh to prevent your old
habits from creeping back in.

Your fitness challenge:

Physical activity is a very important part of a healthy lifestyle.
Think about some easy ways to work more physical activity into
your lifestyle. Review the list below and put a check in the box by
the activities you can commit to doing this week. Get up and get
moving! Strive for thirty to sixty minutes of activity daily.

Helpful Hints for Successful Exercise

- ☐ Take the long way around when walking from one place to another.
- ☐ Take the stairs instead of the elevator.
- ☐ Park farther out in the parking lot at the store or at work.
- ☐ Take five minute walking breaks four to six times each day.
- ☐ Clean your house.
- ☐ Join a gym. If it cost you money, you might be more motivated to do it.
- ☐ Find a walking buddy.
- ☐ Get an accountability partner.

Did You Know?

That you are supposed to drink eight cups of water per day? Water is important for every bodily function. If you don't like plain water, try adding a sugar-free flavor packet to it occasionally. Carry a glass or bottle of water around with you and make yourself sip on it throughout the day. You will be surprised at how quickly you can develop a taste for it.

🍎 **Food Diary**	🙏 **Your Prayer**

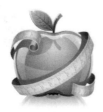

Day 7

The Holy Spirit, Our Helper

God has given you a helper, the Holy Spirit, to guide you through every battle you face, even the battle for your health and weight. As you get older, your metabolism slows down, which means you require less energy to live. If you don't lower your caloric intake as you increase in age, you will gain weight. Therefore, as you get older, controlling your weight gets harder and harder.

This battle can be fought much more easily with God's help, so let's ask for it. Ask the Holy Spirit to be your lifestyle coach. You might wonder, "How do I do that?" You begin with prayer. Pray that God, through His Holy Spirit, will guide you by bringing to light habits you need to change, habits you might not even realize are contributing to your weight problem. Ask Him to help you put Him first in your life instead of food.

Strive to be sensitive to the Holy Spirit's prompting. When you feel guilty about something, it may be more than just your conscience. It may be the Holy Spirit trying to guide you, prompting you to change a habit. If you feel a burden or heaviness about a certain food, habit, or area of your life, start praying about it. Give it to God. Let Him guide you; let Him help you make the changes you need to make to be healthier and lose weight.

Are you a slave to food? Are you turning to food when you should be turning to God? Sins like overeating have a way of enslaving you, controlling you, dominating you, and dictating your actions. Don't be a slave to food and overeating. Put God first in your life, and let Him free you from the things that enslave you.

Every time you feel like you are being controlled or driven by the desire to eat, stop and declare that you are no longer going to let food control you. Ask God to break the hold that food is trying to have on you. Sometimes people use food to fill a void they have in their life, a void that can only be filled by God.

"My food," said Jesus, "is to do the will of him who sent me and to finish his work" (John 4:34).

In this passage, Jesus was referring to the spiritual nourishment you need in your life. This nourishment not only comes from Jesus Christ through Bible study, prayer, and fellowship with other believers; it is the nourishment that comes from doing God's will and helping bring His work of salvation into His world.

Your fitness challenge:
Change your routine today to add at least thirty minutes of physical activity.

Your spiritual challenge:
Praise God for everything that happens to you today.

Don't forget to weigh weekly and plot it on the graph in the front of the book.

Pause now for a moment in God's Word.

Daily Devotion —Day 7

Read Galatians 4:28-5:1. Key verse: Galatians 5:1.

It is for freedom that _____ has set us free. Stand firm, then, and do not let yourself be _____ again by a yoke of slavery.

Sin, such as overeating, has a way of enslaving you, controlling you, and dictating your actions. Jesus can free you from this slavery that keeps you from becoming the person God created you to be.

Have you asked the Holy Spirit to be your lifestyle coach? God is ready to help you. He is just waiting for you to ask. Show Him you are willing to do your part by making sacrifices in your eating habits, and ask Him to come along beside you.

Your nutrition challenge:
Do you skip meals? This week try eating three small meals and two to three snacks per day. You will probably find you consume fewer calories when you are eating more frequently.

Practice eating less. Leave several bites of food on your plate or use a smaller plate to help you decrease your serving sizes.

Team Up With God Today!

🍎 Food Diary	🙏 Your Prayer

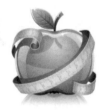

Day 8

So Why Are You Overweight?

So, why are you overweight? For most of you, the answer is going to be because you are taking in more calories than your body needs. Of course, many factors contribute to your weight problem: inactivity, age, illness, or a sudden change in lifestyle. Maybe you went from a job where you were very active to a job where you sit all the time. All of these contribute to your weight, but the fact still remains if you are overweight, you must decrease your calories or increase your activity.

One of the first things you need to do as part of your 40-day journey to a better weight is to make a conscious effort to develop a healthy lifestyle. You can do this by eating healthier and by increasing the amount of physical activity you are getting in the day. Doing these two activities will help you lose weight and keep it off. It will also give you more energy and help you look and feel healthier.

As a general rule, the more you do, the more you will be able to do. Try to exercise every day. How much activity are you currently doing? If you are currently inactive, then get up and get moving!

Start slowly, maybe with five- to ten-minute walks two or three times per day. You need to eventually build up to forty to sixty minutes of physical activity for a minimum of four days per week—ideally five to six days each week. The total time per day is cumulative, so it does not have to be done all at one time.

Physical activity does not have to be in the form of a structured exercise program. You don't have to join a gym to exercise or be physically active. Don't get me wrong, gyms are wonderful; if you can join one, great. Workout facilities are a good way to get productive exercise in a safe environment all at one time. However, don't let the fact that you are not a member of a gym be an excuse to not exercise.

You need to make a conscious effort to build activity into your everyday life, so you can develop a healthy lifestyle. The fact that it is cumulative can help you do things throughout the day to add up to sixty minutes or more of exercise.

I have to admit, I have never been much of a structured exerciser. Every time I start a structured exercise program, it ends up fizzling out with the slightest change in weather or schedule. Lately, I have started going to a gym and getting a good workout at least three to four times per week. Doing so really helps with weight maintenance. I feel better and I look forward to it.

I also find other ways to work activity into my lifestyle. I am a morning person, so I get up early in the morning to have a devotion and prayer time and then spend thirty to sixty minutes cleaning my house. Cleaning house is an excellent way to work physical activity into your life. You can't clean house sitting on the couch or lying in the bed. By cleaning the house throughout the week, it frees up my time on the weekends to do other activities that I love: riding horses, working on projects outside, shopping, or visiting with family.

You need to make exercise and physically activities priorities in your life. In addition to planned exercise time during your day, you need to make a conscious effort to increase your activities throughout the day. This increase can be done by parking further out in parking lots, picking up your pace when walking, and taking the long way around when going to various places throughout the day.

Maintaining an active lifestyle along with regular, scheduled exercise weekly will make losing weight—and keeping it off—easier. It will help you to achieve your weight loss goals. Figure out what works for you. Whether you join a gym and do all your exercising at one time or you exercise in small amounts of activity throughout the day is not important. What is important is that you become more active! So be creative and get moving!

Pause now for a moment in God's Word.

Daily Devotion — Day 8

Read Revelation 22:7-14. Key verses: Revelation 22:12-13.

"Behold, I am coming soon! My _____ is with me, and I will give to everyone according to what He has done. I am the _____ and the _____ the First and the Last, the Beginning and the End."

Think about what you go through to get ready to go somewhere. You take a bath or shower, style your hair, and put on clean clothes, going to great lengths to make sure you are dressed appropriately for the occasion, which only lasts for a short period of time before it's over.

How much time are you spending getting ready for the biggest event of your life—an event which will last an eternity? To do that you must purify yourself from your sinful ways. How do you do that? Spend time daily in the Word seeking God's forgiveness from your sins and going throughout your day in an attitude of prayer and submission to God.

Ask God to reveal any sin in your life that may be getting between you and Him. Then strive to purify yourself from that sin. When you invest your time into getting ready for Christ's return, you are investing in preparation for an event, which will last an eternity. Are you ready?

Your nutrition challenge:
Try to prepare healthy meals and eat at home at least three to four times this week to give you more control of fat and calorie intake.

Food Diary	Your Prayer

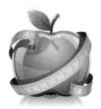

Day 9

Good Versus Bad

When people go on a diet, the first thing they usually do is stop eating all the food they love because they are the "bad" foods. The only problem with this strategy is the foods you love are going to be the foods you crave. After a week or so, you will begin to miss those foods so much you will probably give up on the diet, lose all self-control, and "pig out." As you will discover in *The 40-Day Diet Makeover*, I don't recommend totally restricting the foods you love, just eat less of them or eat them less frequently.

Let me be the bearer of good news. There are no good foods and no bad foods. Yes, some foods are better for you than others, but all foods can be worked into your diet *in moderation*. Most likely, it is not a particular food you are eating that is making you gain weight; it is the amount of food you are eating. Moderation is the key.

Studies have shown that neither a low fat diet nor a low carbohydrate diet is particularly beneficial to your health. What really counts is calories. If you are going to eat something loaded with fat and calories, eating one small serving rather than two large ones is going to be a lot less damaging to your overall caloric intake.

Based on the United States Department of Agriculture (USDA) dietary guidelines for Americans, start making some basic changes in your diet today.

- Eat two to four servings of fruit every day.
- Consume a variety of vegetables. Add more green, yellow, or orange ones and eat fewer of the less colorful, starchy ones.

40

- Most people do not get enough calcium in their diet. Add some low fat, calcium rich food to your diet.

- More of your grains should be whole grains. Look for breads and cereals that will add extra fiber to your diet, especially those that have 100 percent whole wheat. You need twenty-five to thirty-five grams of fiber per day to help regulate bowels. Fiber can also help lower cholesterol and help give you a feeling of fullness, which may help you decrease the amount of food you eat.

- Choose leaner cuts of meat for your protein sources.

- Start limiting the amount of fats, salt, and sugars in your diet.

More details and helpful information can be found on the USDA web site. http://www.usda.gov.

Fat has more calories than anything else you eat. Start decreasing the amount of fat in your diet. Let's look at some easy ways to decrease fat and calories in your diet. For example, what are you eating for breakfast?

TYPICAL BREAKFAST

Sausage and biscuit	430 Calories	29 grams Fat
Medium soft drink	210 Calories	0 grams Fat
TOTAL	640 Calories	29 grams Fat

HEALTHIER BREAKFAST

3/4 cup corn flakes with 2% milk	210 Calories	5 grams Fat
1 banana	120 Calories	0 grams Fat
½ cup orange juice	60 Calories	0 grams Fat
1 slice lt. whole wheat toast w/1 tsp. butter	85 Calories	2.5 grams Fat
TOTAL	475 Calories	7.5 grams Fat

When you make healthier food choices, you may be surprised you can actually have more food with fewer calories and less fat. You don't have to starve to decrease your calories and fat. The same is true for lunch. You can save fat and calories and make your meal healthier by:

- Complementing your sandwich with pretzels or baked chips.

- Using mustard instead of mayonnaise.

- Using whole grain, light bread (40-45 calories per slice compared to 120-160 calories for two slices).

- Eating turkey, ham, grilled chicken, or roast beef rather than bologna, processed meats, or mayonnaise based meat salad.

- Eat only one sandwich instead of two or three.

Eating out has become a way of life for many Americans. Many people cook meals at home fewer than three or four times per week. Without careful planning, your meals away from home could add unwanted fat and calories to your diet, making it almost impossible to get your weight under control.

Making healthier food choices when eating away from home is challenging but not impossible. If you are eating at a fast food restaurant, most offer nutrition guides to help you make informed decisions. When eating with relatives or where nutrition guides are not available, you will want to evaluate the menu choices.

By carefully examining the menu, you can choose foods that are baked, broiled, or grilled, and those that have less added fat and fewer calories. When you pay close attention to the foods you select, you can eat healthy meals away from home and still manage your weight.

TYPICAL FASTFOOD MEAL

4 oz. hamburger & 1 slice of cheese	530 calories	30 grams fat
French fries (large)	610 calories	29 grams fat
large soft drink	310 calories	0 grams fat
TOTAL	1450 calories	59 grams fat

A Healthier Option

grilled chicken on a bun w/mustard, ketchup, pickles (no mayo)	300 calories	6 grams fat
French fries (small)	210 calories	10 grams fat
large diet soft drink	0 calories	0 grams fat
TOTAL	510 calories	16 grams fat

Typical Dessert

candied ice cream dessert	630 calories	23 grams fat

A Healthier Option

vanilla reduced fat ice cream	150 calories	4.5 grams fat

As you can see from the samples above, if you make healthier food choices, you can still eat at your favorite fast food restaurant but save fat and calories. Start thinking about some small changes you can make in your everyday eating habits to cut fat and calories along with increasing your activity level.

The 40-Day Diet Makeover will help you lose weight and keep it off by helping you develop healthy eating habits and a healthier lifestyle, which will last a lifetime. However, as you will probably discover, it is not magic. The book and devotions alone are not going to help you lose weight. The program takes hard work and dedication from you to be effective.

Evaluate Your Diet

1. How many times per week do you eat out (include all three meals)?

_____

2. Do you normally pay attention to how the food is prepared?
____Yes   ____No

3. Write down some changes you can make immediately in your eating habits and food choices to help you decrease your fat and calorie intake.

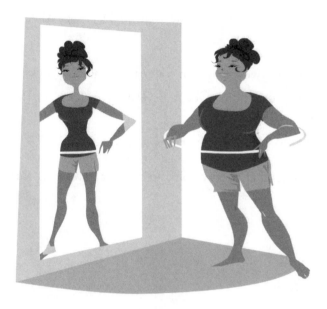

Look at the images above—which side of the mirror are you on? The slim image represents the results of putting time and effort into this program. Committing to *The 40-Day Diet Makeover* one day at a time and making gradual changes in your life will assist you in reaching your goals of permanent weight management and a healthy lifestyle.

Your daily devotions are to help you get into God's Word as well as help reinforce the things you are learning. Take the time to fill in the blanks, work through the activities, and respond to the challenges. Each day builds on the previous day to help you reach the ultimate goals of permanent weight management and healthy lifestyle.

If you do not finish the book, do not make the sacrifices in your diet and exercise program, or don't bother with the devotions or the food diary, then you will probably not attain the healthy body image you would like. To really beat the battle of the bulge and to get the most benefit, you will need to make a daily, hourly, minute-by-minute commitment to this program. You must also be willing to make the permanent changes in your lifestyle.

Remember, this journey is a partnership with God. I am not promising you it will be easy. Just like everything else in life, you will get out of it what you put into it.

I challenge you as you continue your 40-Day Diet Makeover Journey to do the following:

- Make at least two changes in your eating habits or lifestyle per week.
- Have daily devotions. Get into God's Word and invite God to be part of your journey.
- Keep a food diary.

Write two changes that you are going to commit to work on this week:
1.

2.

Did You Know?

The more you do the more you will be able to do. Exercise helps give you energy and keep your joints limber. Work exercise into your life daily.

Pause now for a moment in God's Word.

Daily Devotion — Day 9

Read Hosea 10:12. Key verse: Hosea 10:12.

Sow for yourselves righteousness, reap the fruit of unfailing love, and break up your unplowed ground; for it is time to seek the Lord, until he comes and showers righteousness on you.

Are there areas in your life that are unplowed—areas where you are not letting God have control? God wants you to break up those areas and allow Him in to sow righteousness. When you totally surrender to God, He will transform every corner of your life into glory with His unfailing love and grace. What kind of fruit are you reaping from the seeds you are sowing?

Your nutrition challenge:
Try a new healthy recipe this week.

Your fitness challenge:
Every time you walk somewhere
today, speed up your pace.

Food Diary	Your Prayer

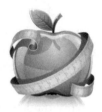

Day 10

Food Fight

Suzy is a thirty-nine-year-old female who weighs approximately 180 pounds and has had a weight problem since she was in her twenties. She has an "I can't" attitude. She looks around and sees nothing but barriers that keep her from being successful at losing weight. She says, "No matter how hard I try, I can't lose weight."

One of the barriers Suzy struggles with is her job. She feels she has no time to cook healthy meals or exercise. This leads to her eating away from home most of the time. Another barrier she faces is food often plays the roles of comforter and stress reliever in her life. Sometimes she feels as if her life centers around food.

Suzy is running late this morning. It has been one of those mornings when everything that could go wrong has gone wrong. As she gets in her car to go to work, she recalls to herself:

Whew, what a morning! The dog got into the garbage and scattered it all over the yard. I was out in my pajamas at 5:30 this morning cleaning it up. The kids were fighting and would not get ready. They almost missed the bus! Joe left for work early, so I had to feed the horses who were not being very cooperative. Now I'm late for work. This is going to be a very bad day.

As Suzy complains about what a horrible day it is going to be, she suddenly notices the food mart where she usually stops on her way to work. She thinks to herself, *I know I'm late, but I sure do need a cappuccino and candy bar. I just don't think I can make it through the day without it, especially as bad as my morning has been.* Before she has time to have second thoughts, she makes a U-turn to go back, even though she is already ten minutes late for work. She runs inside, grabs a big cappuccino and a chocolate candy bar, pays for it very quickly, and rushes back to her car to drive the short distance to work. At the stoplight she takes a bite of the candy bar and a sip of the cappuccino. As the warm liquid slides down her throat, she feels her whole body relax. It immediately changes her whole outlook. She smiles and thinks what a beautiful day. Ahhh. Life is good.

How Does Food Fit into Your Life?

What are your comfort foods and beverages? Obviously, Suzy's comfort foods and beverages are cappuccino and chocolate candy bars. Comfort foods are the foods you use to calm your nerves, to relax when you are uptight and stressed. They are foods which soothe you when you are sick, like chicken noodle soup. Like Suzy, many people use foods to calm them when they are mad or stressed, or to comfort them when they are sick or lonely.

Think about how food fits into your life:

- What foods must you have every day to make your day go right?
- What foods do you crave?
- Is that food controlling you?
- Are you turning to food when you should be turning to God?

God gave us food to enjoy! Many references are included in the Bible to banquets and the enjoyment of food: Jesus feeding the five thousand, Jesus eating with sinners, and the Last Supper. They all center on eating and fellowship. God not only gave us food to enjoy, but He also gave us food for our nourishment. This daily food gives us energy to sustain our life; without it, we would die. Food is not the enemy. It should not control us, it should not be used to comfort us, and it should not take the place of God. How can God be the center of your life if food is?

Let the Holy Spirit be the controlling factor in your life. The Holy Spirit is sent by God to live within you, to convict you, to help you, and to comfort you. Start each morning with prayer, asking God through His Holy Spirit to help you gain control of the food you eat. Ask Him to show you the foods in your life that are controlling you.

Be sensitive to His prompting about your food choices. It may even be something like a diet drink or black coffee that is too important in your life, something not even adding calories but controlling you. You may have to give up that item for a couple of days each week or cut back on it to allow the Holy Spirit to put the food or beverage where it needs to be in your life.

Deuteronomy 14:3-21 defines all the laws the Israelites had to follow in their diet. They followed these laws for a variety of reasons, one being to remind them continuously they were a different and separate people committed to God.

Although we do not have to follow those laws anymore in the New Testament, "Do not call anything impure that God has made clean" (Acts 10:15), we can all learn a lesson of holiness. Holiness is to be carried into all parts of life. The word holy means, "worthy of complete devotion, as one perfect in goodness and righteousness." If we strive for holiness in our life, then we are striving for perfect goodness and righteousness.

As humans, we will never reach perfection, but we can still strive for it. Our health practices, finances, and how we use our leisure time all provide opportunity to put holy living into our daily living.

Christ comes and dwells where there is holiness. For us to experience the abundance life has to offer, we need Christ's presence in our lives. Our body needs to be treated as a temple, a sanctuary, and a place of holiness so we can yoke ourselves with Christ and allow Him to work in us and through us. As you begin to yoke yourself with Christ, you will feel a power over your diet, over your lifestyle, and over your entire life that you have never felt before.

I can do everything through [Christ] who gives me strength (Philippians 4:13).

With Christ in your life, the things that seem impossible, like losing weight and keeping it off, become possible. How does Christ fit into your life? Are you a Christian? Have you accepted Jesus Christ as your Lord and Savior? Have you asked Him into your heart? Do you know beyond a shadow of a doubt that if you died today you would go to heaven?

If you don't, today can be the day of your salvation. Take a moment to say a simple prayer telling God you are a sinner and need His forgiveness.

Then ask Him to come live in your heart. He is waiting for an invitation from you. Nothing is as important as getting your life right with Christ. As you do and strive to make holy living a part of your daily life, He will help you be strong enough to make the changes you need to develop a healthy lifestyle.

Pause now for a moment in God's Word.

Daily Devotion — Day 10

Read 1 John 5:13-20. Key verses: 1 John 5:14-15.

This is the confidence we have in approaching God: that if we ask anything according to his will, he _____ us. And if we know that he _____ us—whatever we ask—we know that we have what we asked of Him.

- Think about how food fits into your life. Is food controlling you?
- Are you addicted to food?
- Is there a certain food or beverage you must have every day to make your day to go right?

Food should not control you. Food should not be the driving force in your life. Ask God for help.

We can approach the throne of God with confidence that He hears our requests and will honor them as long as they line up with His perfect will for our lives. The emphasis here is on *God's will* not our will. Ask God what He wants for you. If you align your prayers to His will, He will listen. He will give you a definite answer. So start praying with confidence. Know He will be there to help you every step of the way as you struggle on your journey. Invite God to be a part of your journey today. He is a great traveling partner.

Your nutrition challenge:
Go a week without eating a particular food
or drinking a certain beverage you think you must have every day.

Food Diary	Your Prayer

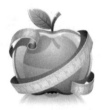

DAY 11

Who Is Going To Win the Battle?

Who is going to win the battle of the bulge? Are you going to win with the help of the Holy Spirit, or are you going to let your flesh win?

Second Timothy 1:7 reminds us,

For God did not give us a spirit of timidity, but a spirit of power, of love and of self-discipline.

Let's explore why you eat the way you do. First, think about your family and the way you were raised. The way a person cooks can be passed from one generation to another. If you were raised by parents or grandparents or great grandparents who fried almost all their meats and put bacon grease or some fat in all the vegetables to season them, then you are probably cooking the same way. The problem is, our lifestyles have changed dramatically over the last 100 years.

Our great-grandparents may have been able to handle an unhealthy diet because most of them were very active and spent a lot of energy to prepare those meals. Back then, if they wanted fried chicken for supper, they had to go to the chicken coop, chase a chicken, kill it, pluck off all the feathers, cut up the chicken, and cook it after they had hauled firewood in to heat up the stove. All this was done by Grandma while Grandpa was plowing the fields with a mule.

The amount of energy your grandparents were expending was far greater than what you spend today on the same fried chicken. Today you buy your chicken already cut up and ready to fry on a stove that heats up with a flick of the switch or even worse, buy it already fried from the local fast food restaurant. While your grandparents were able to use most of the fat and calories for energy, you don't need all the extra fat and calories to do the same chore and so you store them in the form of pounds on your hips. For the most part, you can't eat the way your grandparents ate and still maintain a healthy weight. You have to sacrifice some of those old, unhealthy eating habits for the sake of your health and weight.

You can start by decreasing the amount of fat used in cooking and seasoning your foods. Try to bake, broil, boil, grill, or steam your foods instead of frying them. Begin using beef- or chicken-flavored broth to season your vegetables instead of bacon grease or oil. Start paying attention to what you are eating and cut back on the amount of fried and greasy foods you have. We will go into more detail about this later.

The second factor that contributes to the way you eat is pleasure, which has a huge influence on your eating habits. For instance, maybe you really love the taste of regular ice cream or whole milk and think that low fat milk is just not as good. Or you love your regular soda or sweet tea and can't stand the taste of diet drinks. Sometimes, the answer is to try and just get past the fact it is diet or low fat and decide you are going to like it, training your taste buds to like it.

One of the first changes I made at our house when I started studying nutrition was to switch from whole milk to low fat milk. At first my husband was going to have no part of it. He said that the low fat milk tasted like water, and he couldn't stand to drink it.

One day I decided to pour the low fat milk into the whole milk jug and not tell him. He drank it for a week and could not tell the difference. Of course, when I told him about it, he did not trust me for months. In his opinion, he does not recommend you do this to your family. Every time I would serve something that looked a little different, he would become suspicious and start questioning me. But it was worth it because he eventually started drinking low fat milk and eating healthier.

Many of the low fat or sugar free foods really do taste nearly the same or as good as their counterparts. Give them a chance; be open to trying different things. If you don't like one brand, try a different one. Sometimes that makes a big difference. You can save a lot of calories by switching to diet sodas, sugar free tea, and sugar free flavored drink mixes. Just by drinking one 20 ounce soda (approximately 280 calories) per day more than your body's caloric needs, you could gain sixty pounds per year. Gradually start working the sugar free and low fat versions of foods and beverages into your diet.

The third factor is time. Like Suzy, maybe you don't have time to cook healthy meals, so you end up eating away from home more often than you eat home-cooked meals. Fast foods are a quick way to put on a lot of extra pounds. Super sized food is everywhere. If you're not careful, before long, super sizing is going to super size you!

Time is always going to play an important role in how you eat. You don't have time not to eat healthy meals. With a little forethought and planning, your family can have healthy, home-cooked meals every night with very little effort on your part. Below are just a few tips for you to try:

- Cook on weekends or off days and freeze for busy days during the week.
- Double your recipe when you are cooking soup, spaghetti, or gumbo so you can freeze a batch for later.
- Get up fifteen minutes earlier in the morning so you will have time to put something in the Crock-Pot for supper before you go to work. Purchasing a slow cooker cookbook may be helpful for recipe ideas.
- Keep some healthy, frozen dinners and a bag of salad around for emergency meals.
- Grill extra chicken tenders when grilling on the weekend to put in the freezer for grilled chicken salad during the week.
- Keep some of the quick, all-in-one stir fry meals in the freezer that require very little preparation.
- On a scrap piece of paper, jot down your evening meals for the week. You don't have to have a fancy menu planner to plan healthy meals.

Snacks can also add unwanted fat and calories to your diet. By planning ahead, those snacks can also be made healthier. When you return home from the grocery store, wash your fruits and vegetables, cut them up, and put them in small, individual portion bags. You and your family will be more likely to eat fruits or vegetables for snacks if they are ready to grab and eat. Also, you will be more likely to cook fresh vegetables with your meals if they are already prepared.

You may also find it helpful to buy the single serving, low calorie snacks or divide up snacks like pretzels and baked chips into individual serving sizes to keep for "snack attacks." Even the healthy foods can add unwanted fat and calories if you eat too much of them. The time you spend preparing to eat healthy and planning ahead can make a tremendous difference in the amount of unwanted calories and fat you are consuming.

Daily Devotion — Day 11

Read 1 Corinthians 2:1-9. Key verse: 1 Corinthians 2:9.

"No eye has seen, no ear has heard, no mind has conceived what God has prepared for _____ (your name) who love[s] him."

Are you receiving all that God has in store for you? His dreams for you are so much bigger than you can ever imagine. So let go and let God have more control of your life. Put your future in His hands.

How often do you eat out? _____

What do you usually order? _____

What changes can you make to make it healthier?_____

_____

_____

Your nutrition challenge:

Ask for nutrition guides at all the fast food restaurants where you normally eat so you can make informed decisions about the foods you are eating. Think about how the foods are prepared. Avoid fried foods, super sizes, mayonnaise, cheese, and anything that may add extra fat and calories.

You are loved by God!

🍎 Food Diary	🙏 Your Prayer

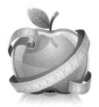

DAY 12

The Road to Success

Part of the plan of attack to eating healthy meals is to become aware of exactly how much you are eating each day. Your increased awareness will help you address those areas that need improvement. Pay closer attention to the food you eat. This means being aware of the amount of fat and calories you put in your mouth.

Remember Suzy? She needed help. She was overweight, overworked, and under-motivated. In her desperation to get her weight under control, she enrolled in a *40-Day Diet Makeover* class being taught at her local church. She knew she needed to do something to get her life under control. One of the first things Suzy learned was that small changes reap lasting rewards. What Suzy focused on was making one small permanent change in her diet or lifestyle at a time. She found she could handle changing one thing at a time, and each change she made—or new habit she started—built on the previous change.

First, Suzy started decreasing her serving sizes. She liked making this change because it allowed her to eat what she normally ate, but by eating less, she was decreasing her total calorie intake. As she grew accustomed to eating less, she seemed to be getting full quicker. Her stomach seemed to be shrinking. She really didn't miss the food she was not eating and was not feeling hungry after she left the table.

After a few weeks of decreasing her serving sizes, Suzy's devotional time and work in her *40-Day Diet Makeover* journal led her to take another step in changing her eating habits. She realized she was taking in too many sweets. She drank sweet tea, sweetened beverage drinks, punch, and regular soda. All added sugar and empty calories to her diet. She decided she was tired of wasting her calories on sweetened beverages, so she switched to unsweetened tea, sugar free sweetened beverages, and diet drinks. Once Suzy's taste buds got used to the taste of diet and sugar free drinks, she didn't even miss the sweetened variety.

When she was ready to go one step further with her sweet intake, she started limiting the amount of other sweets such as candies, cookies, and pies. Suzy realized these baked sweets are usually loaded with empty, unwanted calories and fat. Although she has not totally cut those out, she has significantly decreased the frequency and the amount of sweets she was eating. By cutting back on the amount of sugar in her diet and decreasing her serving sizes, she was beginning to lose weight.

Suzy felt as though she were making progress and made another change to her lifestyle by decreasing her intake of fast foods. Instead of eating out every day for lunch and at least three to four nights a week, Suzy began taking her lunch to work and only ate out one to two nights per week. With the new routine, she was planning her meals and cooking more at home. This really helped her save calories and lose even more weight. Up to this point, she had never realized how many extra calories she was taking in from restaurant meals or how much money she was spending on them.

With her new weight loss, Suzy began to feel better. She had more energy, so she decided it was time to start getting more daily physical activity. She began getting up thirty minutes earlier so she had time for devotions plus time to walk at least fifteen to twenty minutes in the morning before work. Since she brought her lunch to work now, she had time to walk with her friends during the last part of her lunch hour. She also tried to stop at the gym on her way home from work for a little workout. The increased activity really helped her maintain her weight loss.

Six months into the program, Suzy has lost forty pounds and is doing great. Her whole outlook on life has changed. She now has an "I can" rather than an "I can't" attitude. With Suzy making one small change at a time, she gradually developed a healthy lifestyle. Suzy's new behavior will help her reap the rewards of being able to maintain her weight loss.

Like Suzy, if you start today implementing small, gradual changes in your diet and lifestyle, you will find you will be able to lose weight and keep it off.

Here are some small changes you can easily make:

- Take your time when you eat. It takes twenty minutes for your brain to tell your stomach you're full. You can eat a lot of food in twenty minutes. Chew your food slowly, put your fork down between bites, and stop eating before you feel full.

- Fill half your plate with salad and/or vegetables, with only small servings of meat, bread, and desserts. Salad and vegetables have fewer calories and are more nutrient rich than meats, breads, and starches.

- Set a goal to lose one to two pounds per week. Losing weight too quickly is dangerous and usually results in disaster. Diets that promote quick weight loss usually change your eating habits drastically without promoting any lifestyle change. Consequently, when you get off the diet and go back to eating the way you used to eat, you end up gaining the weight back plus an extra five to ten pounds. If you implement gradual lifestyle changes, your weight loss may be slower, but it will be long-lasting.

- Keeping a food diary is a very helpful tool for weight management. The extra time you take doing it will reap enduring rewards.

- Be realistic; don't be tricked by Hollywood images. Many of those visible in society have access to personal trainers and chefs, plenty of extra time, cosmetic surgery, and photo touch-ups.

Pause now for a moment in God's Word.

Daily Devotion — Day 12

Read Acts 10:1-15. Key verses: Acts 10:14-15.

"Surely not, Lord!" Peter replied. "I have never eaten anything impure or unclean." The voice spoke to him a second time, "Do not call anything _____ that God has made _____."

God gave us food to nourish us, to sustain our life and for us to enjoy. Food is not our enemy! There is no good food versus bad food. All food can fit into your life! The key is moderation! It is not what you eat but how much you eat that makes the food bad for you.

Your nutrition challenge:
Work your favorite foods into your diet in moderation!

Your fitness challenge:
Walk three-fourths of a mile today.

🍎 **Food Diary**	🙏 **Your Prayer**

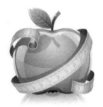

DAY 13

Step By Step

Something most of us struggle with is keeping our homes clean and livable. I am no exception. Keeping my house clean can sometimes be overwhelming, especially when all three of my boys are home messing it up as fast as I clean. More often than I would like to admit, the mess in my house gets out of control with every room in total chaos. I can handle a mess for a little while, but sooner or later I reach my limit. When I do, you better stay out of my way because I am going to put everyone in my path to work until every last room is spotless.

If I clean like my friend cleans, the chore will take me forever. I will probably wind up getting frustrated and quit halfway through. My friend is easily distracted. She will start cleaning the bedroom, notice that the kids have left dirty dishes there, causing her to leave her task of cleaning up the bedroom to take the plates and cups to the kitchen.

There she notices the sink is full of dirty dishes and starts washing them. Then the phone rings, so she leaves the sink of dishes to answer the phone. While she is on the phone, she notices the mail scattered all over the counter, so she starts sorting through it but has to leave it when one of the kids wants her to come help them put a light bulb in the bathroom. Once she gets the light bulb replaced, she notices the tub needs cleaning and starts cleaning it. And so on. Four hours later she looks around to find a bedroom still dirty, a sink half full of dirty dishes, and mail she has not finished sorting. She feels completely defeated and ready to quit.

When I clean, I try to make myself focus on one small area at a time, and clean and organize it completely before moving on to the next task—even if it means I have to pile all the dirty clothes and dishes in the hall while I finish cleaning the bedroom. I am much more productive if I can stay in one area and completely finish it before moving on to the next job. plus it gives me such a feeling of victory and satisfaction when I get one room completely cleaned. It motivates me to press on and finish the rest of the house.

The same concept can be used to help you reach your weight loss goals. If you concentrate on taking it step by step, changing one thing at a time in your diet or lifestyle, you will not feel overwhelmed and be as tempted to throw in the towel. Don't fool yourself into thinking the weight—which took years to gain—is going to come off in two months. Set small, realistic goals that are achievable. If you can reach one small goal at a time, you will be able to celebrate your success at each step of the way and be motivated to strive toward the next goal.

Deciphering Nutrition Labels

Nutrition labels are put on food products to aid in making informed decisions about the foods we eat. However, they can be very confusing if you don't know how to read them. When looking at a food label, focus on three main things:

- Serving Size
- Calories (per serving)
- Total Fat (grams per serving)

Tortilla Chips

Serving Size	1 package
Servings Per Container	1
Calories	260
Total Fat	13g
Saturated Fat	2g
Trans Fat	0g
Cholesterol	less than 5mg
Sodium	350mg
Total Carbohydrates	31g
Dietary Fiber	2g
Sugars	2g
Protein	4g

The first thing you want to look at is *serving size*. For example, if the label says the serving size is one cookie, then the first thing you have to decide is whether one cookie is enough to fill you up or satisfy you. If one cookie is big, then it might be enough to satisfy you. But if one cookie is quite small, then it won't be enough to satisfy you and if the calorie count is high, it will not be a good choice.

Serving sizes are very important. Often people will think they are eating a healthy food because they are eating a low fat product. However, when they eat two to three servings of the low fat food, they end up consuming more fat and calories than they would get from one serving of another food.

For example, one serving of pretzels will give you about 100 calories, a good choice for a snack. However, if you eat four servings at one time, then you will get 400 calories from that snack. Not good. So serving size is very important!

The second thing you want to look at is *calories per serving*. The number of calories per serving can be helpful to you if you are trying to conserve your calories. It can also be very helpful in comparing foods. For example, if you are comparing breads, one bread might have 140 calories in two slices, while the other bread only has 90 calories in two slices. If you choose the one with 90 calories per two slices, then you will be saving 50 calories with every sandwich you eat. It's wise to compare food items and choose the one that will give you the least number of calories per serving without greatly compromising taste and quality.

The third thing you want to look for on the nutrition label is the *number of grams of fat per serving*. Fat has more calories than any other nutrient. If you limit the grams of fat you are eating, you will be decreasing your total calorie intake. We will go into more details later about fats in your diet, but as a general rule, you should try to choose snacks that will give you no more than four to six grams of fat per serving. Gather a few products from your own pantry and practice reading their nutrition labels.

Compare Nutrition Labels to Choose Healthier Foods

Sweet Cracker Sticks   Tortilla Chips

Serving Size: 14 sticks ← → Serving Size: 1 package

Servings Per Container: about 12   Servings Per Container: 1

Calories 130 ← → Calories 260

Total Fat 2.5g ← → Total Fat 13g

Saturated Fat 0.5g   Saturated Fat 2g

Polyunsaturated Fat 0g   Trans Fat 0g

Monounsaturated Fat 1g   Cholesterol less than 5mg

Cholesterol 0mg   Sodium 350mg

Sodium 170mg   Total Carbohydrate 31g

Total Carbohydrate 24g   Dietary Fiber 2g

Dietary Fiber less than 1g   Sugars 2g

Sugars 9g   Protein 4g

Protein 2g

Choose healthier snacks by comparing the food labels. If the two snacks above were your next choices for a snack, which one would be the better choice? You could save 130 calories and 10.5 grams of fat by choosing the Sweet Crackers over the Tortilla Chips.

Your nutrition challenge:
Pay closer attention to the food you are putting in your mouth.

Your fitness challenge:
Ask a friend to exercise with you today.

Pause now for a moment in God's Word.

Daily Devotion — Day 13

Read Psalm 25:1-15. Key verses: Psalm 25:4-5.

Show me your _____, O Lord, teach me your paths; guide me in your _____ and teach me, for you are _____ my _____, and my _____ is in you all day long.

Did You Know?

Our God is a God of second chances. He is patient and kind as He teaches us His ways and guides our steps. When we get off track and venture out on our own, He will draw us back to Him and be there waiting for us. Like a Father waiting for a wayward child to come home, God will always take us back. When we come back asking for forgiveness, He will give us as many second chances as it takes to keep us in His grasp.

Test your skills at reading food labels. Get a snack food from your cabinet:

- What is the serving size? _____
- How many servings per container? _____
- How many calories per serving? _____
- How much fat per serving? _____ grams
- Total carbohydrates? _____ grams
- Dietary fiber? _____ grams
- Protein? _____ grams

The more informed you are about the foods you are eating, the better choices you can make!

🍎 Food Diary	🙏 Your Prayer

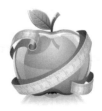

Day 14

Calorie Counting

Over and over again, clients come to my office wanting a specific calorie level diet with menus to help them with weight management. They think if someone will just give them a menu, telling them what to eat with exact serving sizes, it will solve all their weight problems. Sounds good, doesn't it? In a fantasy world this concept would work perfectly, because I could give the client a set of menus that would magically contain all the foods they prefer. The client could take them home to their full-time cook, who would cook exactly what is on the menus for each meal, and the client would always be at home to eat those meals as they are prepared.

However, in the real world, most of us do not have a full-time cook, everyone has different food preferences, and our schedules are not the same every day. Therefore, we can't be that structured with our eating habits. Remember, *The 40 Day Diet Makeover* is not a diet; it is a lifestyle. Following a calorie controlled diet for a lifetime is not practical, and this dietitian does not recommend it for long-term use.

Nevertheless, I do think it is important to have a concept of approximately how many calories you need each day to help promote weight loss and to help you pay more attention to exactly how much you should be eating. How many calories per day are you currently eating? Do you have a clue?

Most of you probably have no idea; you eat when you are hungry, paying little attention to what or how much you are eating. Calorie counting, along with food journaling, can be a very helpful tool to get you on the track of eating less, monitoring what you are eating, and helping you not to cheat.

The amount of energy your body needs every day to function depends on your size and activity level. Calories are your body's energy source. When it comes to calorie counting and nutrition, many helpful resources are right at your fingertips. A good example is MyPyramid.gov. This website is set up by the USDA to help give you good, reliable nutrition information. It will provide you with an estimate for recommended calories per day and number of servings from each food group for your specific calorie level. You may need to adjust these calories up or down as you monitor your weight loss progress.

There are 3,500 calories in one pound. You must decrease your calories by 500 calories a day to lose one pound per week. Therefore, if you are currently eating 2,000 calories per day, you will need to subtract five hundred calories, which will give you 1,500 calories a day for weight loss.

This is only an estimate of your calorie needs. Remember, everyone is different. As I stated earlier, we don't all fit into the same box. The way your body handles calories is going to be totally different from the way someone else's handles calories.

You may eat the exact number of calories that your friend—who is about your size—eats, and she loses weight while your weight stays the same. Therefore, your calorie needs have to be based on the way your body handles energy. This has to be determined by trial and error. So where do you start? First you need to estimate the approximate number of calories you need per day. See the guidelines below.

Estimated Daily Calories

The number of calories needed daily depends upon age, size, and activity level. Calories are your body's main source of energy. As a general rule, men need 2,000-2,500 calories per day. Women need 1,500-1,800 calories per day.

Individualize your calorie needs by monitoring weight loss and adjusting calorie level to achieve a weight loss of one to two pounds per week. Calorie counting is a useful tool to help you realize how many calories a day you need to be eating. However, I do not recommend it for a long period of time because it is so restrictive. Remember *The 40-Day Diet Makeover* incorporates eating habits that will last a lifetime.

As I stated earlier, your calorie needs should be individualized based on the way your body handles energy. Start out with the highest number of calories you think you could eat and still lose weight. Stay at that level for a week or so. Monitor your weight and make adjustments up or down to achieve a weight loss of one to two pounds per week.

The forms and information on the following pages should help guide you through the calorie counting process. Included is a guide for planning calorie controlled diets, a food guide, and a menu planning worksheet. If you would like to try a calorie controlled diet for a short period of time, these guides can be used to plan your own calorie specific menus.

WARNING: *The calorie counting information below can be complicated; if you want to keep your journey to a healthier weight simple, skip over to the day 14 devotion.*

Guide for Planning Calorie Controlled Diets

	2,000 calories	1800 calories	1500 calories	1200 calories
BREAKFAST				
Juice/Fruit	1	1	1	1
Starch/Bread	2	2	2	1
Meat	1	1	1	0
Bacon/Fat	2	1	1	1
Skim Milk	1	1	1	1
LUNCH				
Meat - Med Fat	3	3	2	2
Starch/Bread	3	2	2	1
Vegetable	2	2	2	2
Fruit	1	1	1	1
Fat	1	1	1	1
SUPPER				
Meat - Med Fat	3	3	2	2
Starch/Bread	3	3	2	1
Vegetable	3	3	2	3
Fruit	1	1	1	1
Fat	1	1	1	1
SNACK				
Bread or Skim Milk	2	1	1	1
Fruit	1	1	1	1

To plan a calorie controlled diet using the previous table, decide on how many calories you wish to consume and then take the numbers from the appropriate, put them in the worksheet below, and plan your meals.

The 40-Day Diet Makeover Menu Planning Worksheet

Calories Per Day: _____

# of SERV.	FOOD GROUP	MENU
		BREAKFAST
	Juice/Fruit	
	Starch/Bread	
	Meat	
	Bacon/Fat	
	Skim Milk	
		LUNCH
	Meat - Med Fat	
	Starch/Bread	
	Vegetable	
	Fruit	
	Fat	
		SUPPER
	Meat - Med Fat	
	Starch/Bread	
	Vegetable	
	Fruit	
	Fat	
		SNACK
	Bread or Milk	
	Fruit	

The Food Guide below is broken up into the food groups. It provides you with the serving sizes for a variety of foods in each food group. Each serving size is equal to one serving. Therefore, if your Menu Planning Worksheet says you can have two servings of bread or starch then you can look in the bread or starch section of the Food Guide below and choose two items, such as one slice of toast and one-half cup oatmeal. Or you can choose one item and have two servings of it such as one cup of oatmeal. Therefore, the Menu Planning Worksheet will help you develop calorie-controlled menus specific to your likes and dislikes.

Food Guide
Serving Sizes & Calories / Serving

STARCH/BREAD:
One serving of bread or starch = 80 calories, 15 grams carbohydrates, 3 grams of protein, and 0-1 gram of fat.

BREAD

1 slice	bread
2 slices	reduced calorie
1/2	hot dog/hamburger bun
1	pancake
1	small roll
1	tortilla
2" sq.	cornbread
1 small	biscuit
1/2	4oz ounce bagel

CEREAL / GRAINS

1/2 cup	bran cereal
1/2 cup	grits or oatmeal
3/4 cup	unsweetened cereal
1/3 cup	pasta (cooked)
1/3 cup	rice (cooked)

STARCHY VEGETABLES

1/3 cup	baked beans
1/2 cup	corn
1/2 cup	peas
2/3 cup	Lima beans
1/2 cup	potatoes
1/2	potato (medium)
1 cup	French fries

CRACKERS / SNACKS

8	animal crackers
3 cups	low fat popcorn
6	Saltine crackers
15-20	baked chips

FRUITS

One serving of fruit = 60 calories and
15 grams of carbohydrates.

1 small	apple		3/4 cup	fresh pineapple
1/2 cup	applesauce		1/2 cup	canned pineapple
1 small	banana		2 Tbl.	raisins
3/4 cup	blueberries		1 1/4 cups	strawberries
1 cup	cantaloupe		1 1/4 cups	watermelon
2 med.	figs		1/2 cup	apple juice
1/2 cup	fruit cocktail		1/3 cup	cranberry juice
1/2	grapefruit		1/3 cup	grape juice
17	grapes		1/2 cup	orange juice
1 Small	orange		1/2 cup	pineapple juice
1 med.	peach		1/3 cup	prune juice
1/2 lg.	pear		1/2 cup	canned peaches/pears

MILK

Milk and dairy products:
calories and fat vary according to choices.

	Carbs	Protein	Fat	Calories
Fat Free / Skim	12 grams	8 grams	0-3 grams	90
Reduced Fat (2%)	12 grams	8 grams	5 grams	120
Whole	12 grams	8 grams	8 grams	150

1 cup	milk
1 cup	buttermilk
½ cup	evaporated milk
3/4-1 cup	yogurt

VEGETABLES

One serving of vegetables = 25 calories,
5 grams carbohydrates, 2 grams protein, 0 grams fat.

Vegetables: one serving = 1/2 cup cooked or 1 cup raw

artichoke hearts	greens (turnip, collard, kale, mustard)
asparagus	mushrooms
green beans	okra
beets	onion
broccoli	peppers (all varieties)
Brussel sprouts	radishes
cabbage	salad greens (lettuce, spinach, Romaine)
carrots	sauerkraut
cauliflower	spinach
celery	summer squash
cucumber	water chestnuts
eggplant	zucchini

MEATS

Meats: Calories and Fat Vary According to Choices.

	Carbs	Protein	Fat	Calories/Ounce
Very lean	0 grams	7 grams	0-1 grams	35
Lean	0 grams	7 grams	3 grams	55
Med. Fat	0 grams	7 grams	5 grams	75
High Fat	0 grams	7 grams	8 grams	100

Very Lean Meats

1 ounce	Chicken (white meat, no skin)
1 ounce	Cornish hen (no skin)
1 ounce	Fish: fresh or frozen cod, flounder, haddock, halibut, trout, smoked salmon, fresh or canned (in water), tuna
1 ounce	Shellfish: clams, crab, lobster, scallops, shrimp, imitation
1 ounce	Game: duck, pheasant (no skin), venison
1 ounce	Sandwich meat: turkey, ham, or beef
1 ounce	Fat free or low fat hot dogs (with 1 gram of fat per serving)
1 ounce	Low fat sausage (1 gram or less of fat per serving)

1 ounce	cheese with 1 gram fat or less per ounce
1/4 cup	cottage cheese (or 1 oz. fat free cheese)
2	egg whites
1/4 Cup	egg substitutes (plain)

Count the Following as I Lean Meat and I Starch:
| 1/2 Cup | Dried beans, peas, lentils (cooked) |

Lean Meats and Substitutes
1 ounce	Beef: USDA select or choice grades of lean beef (trimmed of fat): round, sirloin, flank steak, tenderloin, roast (rib, chuck, rump), steak, (T-bone, porterhouse, cubed), ground round
1 ounce	Pork: lean pork: fresh, canned, cured, boiled ham; Canadian bacon, tenderloin, center loin chop
1 ounce	Lamb: roast, chop, leg
1 ounce	Veal: lean, chop roast
1 ounce	Poultry: chicken (white meat with skin), turkey (dark meat, no skin), domestic duck or goose (well-drained of fat, no skin)
1 ounce	Fish: herring (uncreamed or smoked)
6 medium	Oysters
1 ounce	Fish: salmon (fresh or canned), catfish, tuna (canned in oil, drained)
1 ounce	Game: goose (no skin), rabbit
1/4 cup	cottage cheese (4.5% fat)
2 Tbl.	grated parmesan
1 ounce	cheese (with three grams of fat or less per ounce)
1-1/2 oz.	hot dogs (with three grams of fat or less per ounce)
1 ounce	processed sandwich meat (with three grams of fat or less per ounce): turkey, pastrami, kielbasa

Medium Fat Meat and Substitutes List
1 ounce	Beef: most beef products fall into this category (ground, meat-loaf, corned, short ribs (prime grades trimmed of fat), prime rib
1 ounce	Pork: top loin, chop, Boston butt, cutlet
1 ounce	Poultry: chicken (dark meat with skin), ground turkey, ground chicken, fried chicken (with skin)
1 ounce	Fish: any fried fish product

1 ounce	Cheese: any cheese (with five grams of fat or less per ounce) Mozzarella cheese
1	egg
1 ounce	sausage (with five grams of fat or less per ounce)

High Fat Meat and Substitutes List

1 ounce	Pork: spare ribs, ground, sausage
1 ounce	Cheese: All regular cheese: American, cheddar, Monterey Jack, Swiss
1 ounce	Processed sandwich meats: bologna, pimento loaf, salami (with eight grams of fat or less per ounce)
1 ounce	Sausage: bratwurst, Italian, knockwurst, Polish, smoked
1 ounce	Hot dogs: chicken or turkey
3 slices	bacon
1 Tbl.	peanut butter

Count the Following Item as I High Fat & I Fat Exchange

1	Hot dog: beef, pork, or combination

FATS

One serving of fat = 5 grams of fat and 45 calories.

Monounsaturated Fat (the best choice)

2 Tbl.	medium avocado
1 tsp.	Oil: canola, olive, peanut
8	black ripe olives
10 lge.	green stuffed olives
6	almonds, cashews
6	mixed nuts
10	peanuts
4 halves	pecans
1/2 Tbl.	peanut butter
1 Tbl.	sesame seeds

Polyunsaturated Fat

1 tsp.	Margarine: stick, tub, squeeze
1 Tbl.	low fat spread

1 tsp.	regular mayonnaise
1 Tbl.	reduced fat mayonnaise
4 halves	Nuts: walnuts, English
1 tsp.	Oil: corn, safflower, soybean
1 Tbl.	regular salad dressing
2 Tbl.	reduced fat salad dressing
1 Tbl.	Seeds: pumpkin, sunflower

Saturated Fat (most unhealthy fat)

1 slice	Bacon: cooked
1 tsp.	Bacon: grease
1 tsp.	Butter: stick
2 tsp.	Butter: whipped
1 Tbl.	Butter: reduced fat
2 Tbl.s	Coconut: sweetened, shredded
2 Tbl.	Cream: half & half
1 Tbl.	Regular cream cheese
1-1/2 Tbl.	Reduced fat cream cheese
2 Tbl.	Regular sour cream
3 Tbl.	Reduced fat sour cream
1 tsp.	Shortening or lard

Example of a Three-Day
1500 Calorie Meal Plan

BREAKFAST — Day I

# Serv.	Food Group	Menu
1	Fruit	4 oz orange juice
2	Starch/Bread	2 slices light toast* 1/2 cup oatmeal
1	Meat	1 egg
1	Fat	1 tsp. butter
1	Milk	1 cup skim milk

*Note: * 2 slices light bread = 1 bread*

LUNCH — Day I

# Serv.	Food Group	Menu
2	Meat	2 oz. ham
2	Starch/Bread	2 slices light bread 1 oz. baked chips
2	Vegetables	salad & 4 oz V8 juice
1	Fruit	15 grapes
1	Fat	1 Tbl. diet dressing (mustard and pickles on sandwich) sugar-free beverage or water

SUPPER — Day I

# Serv.	Food Group	Menu
2	Meat	2 oz. grilled chicken
2	Starch/Bread	1 small baked potato and 1 roll
2	Vegetables	1/2 cup broccoli 1/2 cup green beans
1	Fruit	1/2 cup peaches in sugar-free Jello
1	Fat	3 Tbl. low fat sour cream sugar-free beverage, water, or free foods

SNACK — Day I

# Serv.	Food Group	Menu
1	Bread/Milk	1 cup low fat fruit yogurt
1	Fruit	1 bottle water

MENU DAY 2

BREAKFAST — Day 2

# Serv.	Food Group	Menu
1	Fruit	1-1/4 cup strawberries
2	Starch/Bread	2 pancakes with light syrup
1	Meat	1 turkey sausage
1	Fat	1 Tbl. low fat margarine
1	Milk	1 cup skim milk

LUNCH — Day 2

# Serv.	Food Group	Menu
2	Meat	2 turkey rolls with 1 oz. turkey 1 low fat cheese (also counts as 1 fat)
2	Starch/Bread	2 small flour tortillas
2	Vegetables	onion, bell pepper, lettuce
1	Fruit	1 apple
1	Fat	(included above in cheese)
		sugar-free beverage or water

SUPPER — Day 2

# Serv.	Food Group	Menu
2	Meat	2 oz. tuna on
2	Starch/Bread	2 slices light bread 1 small corn on the cob
2	Vegetables	1 cup steamed vegetables
1	Fruit	1/2 cup juice
1	Fat	1 Tbl. low fat mayonnaise
		sugar-free beverage or water

SNACK — Day 2

# Serv.	Food Group	Menu
1	Bread or Milk	1/2 cup light ice cream with fruit topping
1	Fruit	

MENU DAY 3

BREAKFAST — Day 3

# Serv.	Food Group	Menu
1	Fruit	1 small banana
2	Starch/Bread	3/4 cup unsweetened cereal 1 slice toast
1	Meat	1 egg
1	Fat	1 slice bacon
1	Milk	1 cup skim milk

LUNCH — Day 3

# Serv.	Food Group	Menu
2	Meat	1 small hamburger with ketchup, mustard, pickles
2	Starches/Bread	1 small hamburger bun
2	Vegetables	1/2 cup steamed mixed vegetables 1 small salad
1	Fruit	1 small orange
1	Fat	2 Tbl. light salad dressing
		sugar-free beverage or water

SUPPER — Day 3

# Serv.	Food Group	Menu
2	Meat	1 BBQ pork chop
2	Starch/Bread	1 slice corn bread 1/2 cup peas
2	Vegetables	1 cup steamed cabbage
1	Fruit	1/2 cup pineapple
1	Fat	1 tsp. margarine on vegetables
		sugar-free beverage or water

SNACK — Day 3

# Serv.	Food Group	Menu
1	Bread or Milk	1 bag snack size popcorn
1	Fruit	1 small fruit cup with light syrup
		1 bottle water

Meal planning can be time consuming but very helpful when you are trying to see exactly how much food you should be eating and to prevent overeating. It is also helpful to plan your menu, then build your grocery list based on your menu. When you go to the grocery store, only purchase the foods on your list. This will help keep you from overspending and impulse buying.

As a reminder, this dietitian does not recommend you follow a strict calorie controlled diet or use counting calories as a way of life. However, using calorie counting for a short period of time can be useful.

RECIPE CORNER

Low Fat Gravy
For Chicken, Beef, or Deer Steak

1 to 2 cans of low fat, low sodium cream of mushroom soup
1 can of low sodium beef broth soup

Saute seasoned meat in a skillet, then drain on a paper towel. Pour excess grease from skillet. Pour soups into the skillet. With a wire whisk, stir until well mixed; bring to boil then simmer until thick. Pour over sautéed chicken, lean beef, or deer steak in a Dutch oven or casserole dish. Cover and cook at 275° for 2 to 3 hours. You may increase the oven temperature and decrease the cooking time if desired.

Pause now for a moment in God's Word.

Daily Devotion — Day 14

Read Ecclesiastes 3:1-14. Key verse: Ecclesiastes 3:1.

There is a _____ for everything, and a season for every _____ under heaven.

Time. There is never enough time! Who has time to cook or eat in a healthy way? Or exercise? Satan is the author of chaos and confusion. He loves it when we are so busy our world is spinning out of control. That is why you need to take control in the midst of the chaos by getting organized and using your time wisely.

- Think about a typical day in your world. What do you spend most of your time doing?

- What is wasting your time?

- What crumbs of time could you use more wisely?

- Can you change your schedule to save thirty minutes or more of wasted time per day?

- By planning ahead you can use your time more efficiently and set aside time to cook healthy meals and to exercise.

- Start each day by praying God will help you make the most of the crumbs of time you have to help you cook and eat healthier and to exercise.

Your spiritual challenge:
Try getting up thirty minutes earlier each day for quiet time with God.

Food Diary	**Your Prayer**

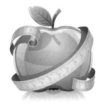

DAY 15

Self-Control—God Control

Look up 1 Peter 5:8 and fill in the blanks.

Be self-controlled and _____. Your enemy the _____ prowls around like a roaring lion looking for someone to devour.

Self-control—some have it, others want it, and we all need it. Lack of self-control can get you in a ton of trouble. It may cause you to spend more than your means, charge on credit cards, and slide into debt. It may cause you to abuse your time, spending more time playing or sleeping than working or serving God. Or it may cause you to drink or eat too much. If you have a lack of self-control in your life, you need to act as Peter suggests in 1 Peter 5:6.

Humble yourselves, therefore, under God's mighty hand, that he may lift you up in due time.

When you humbly confess your weaknesses before God and ask for His help, He will help you. He can help you develop self-control in your life. Start today letting your life be God controlled. Through Him, you can find real self-control. Let God transform your mind. How do you do this? Get into God's Word daily, pray continuously, and fellowship with fellow believers. If you are not in a church, consider joining one.

We cannot stand against Satan on our own. He is powerful but can be defeated by the Master, our Lord and Savior Jesus Christ. Allow God to control every aspect of your life and to develop the self-control you need to lose weight and keep it off.

Get Up and Get Moving

Being physically active also takes self-control and should be an integral part of a healthy lifestyle. Evaluate your current level of activity. Make every attempt to gradually increase your activity. Below are some tips to help you be more active:

- Hide the remote so you have to get up to change the television channel.
- Park as far away from the store as possible when going shopping.
- Clean your house daily.
- Mow your yard with a push mower.
- When exercising, start slowly—maybe five to ten minutes per hour or fifteen to twenty minutes per day, then gradually increase to forty to sixty minutes or more daily.

Remember, the more you do, the more you will be able to do.

Your fitness challenge:
Exercise is an important part of this program.
Find time to fit exercise into your busy schedule.
Exercise thirty to forty minutes daily.

Did You Know?

An isolated Christian is a paralyzed Christian. You need to be active in your local church. Fellowship with other believers. Carve out time from your busy schedule to spend worshiping with your bothers and sisters in Christ.

Pause now for a moment in God's Word.

Daily Devotion — Day 15

Read Psalm 20:4-9. Key verse: Psalm 20:4.

May He give you the desire of your heart and make all your plans succeed.

When the desires of your heart center on Jesus and His perfect will, then He will help direct your path toward success. Pray before planning your day, your week, or your life. He wants your plans to succeed, but they must be His will, not yours.

Your nutrition challenge:

Below are some tips to help you achieve success on your
journey to weight loss. Put a check by the things you will commit
to incorporate into your busy lifestyle to help you
and your family eat healthier.

- ☐ Cook ahead on weekends or days off and freeze meals for busy days.
- ☐ Use your Crock-Pot.
- ☐ Plan your menus before you go grocery shopping.
- ☐ Prepare foods in the morning or the night before for easy meal preparation.
- ☐ Wash and cut up fruits and vegetables as soon as they are purchased.
- ☐ Cook meats in bulk to be used in soups, sauces, and casseroles.
- ☐ Buy healthy, frozen meals for use in emergencies.
- ☐ Avoid frying your foods.
- ☐ Decrease the number of times you eat out—including lunch—to one-third of what you are currently doing.

Failure To Plan Is Planning To Fail!

Food Diary	**Your Prayer**

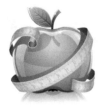

DAY 16

The War Within

What are your struggles? What are the battles you fight in your life? What does your enemy look like? Your conflicts can take on many different shapes and forms. They change from day to day and year to year. They may be in the form of everyday problems with your kids, spouse, relatives, or a boss. It may be a battle with a temporary illness, or it may be a more long-term battle with finances. Maybe you have dug a hole of financial debt you can't seem to get out of. You may have a fight with time management—you never have enough hours in the day to accomplish everything that needs to be done. For some of you it is laziness, depression, an addiction to drugs, or alcohol. For many people the battle is with food.

God uses food for our nourishment and enjoyment. Satan wants us to abuse food by stuffing ourselves, which is called gluttony. Good nutrition and a healthy lifestyle reap good health, whereas poor nutrition and an unhealthy lifestyle reap destruction—chronic diseases and illnesses. Satan knows you are vulnerable when it comes to food; he knows the cracks in your foundation. Don't think he won't attack every chance he gets. You must prepare for battle.

How Do You Prepare for Battle?

You need to start each day by putting on the full armor of God. You can do this by praying the prayer below based on Ephesians 6:11-18. Make this prayer a part of your daily devotion. There is power in Scripture. When you take Scripture and apply it to your life, it gives you the ability to invoke God's power in your life in a new way. Ephesians 6:11-18 is one of the most powerful defenses we have against Satan's attacks. Try applying these verses to your life daily and watch your world turn around.

A paraphrase of Ephesians 6:11–18:

Put on the full armor of God so you can take your stand against the devil's schemes. For our struggle is not against flesh and blood, but against the rulers, against the authorities, against the powers of this dark world. Therefore, put on the full armor of God so when you are attacked you can stand firm.

Prayer:

Lord, today I buckle the belt of truth around my waist. I put on the breastplate of righteousness, and I have my feet fitted for readiness, which comes from the gospel of peace. I take up the shield of faith, with which I can extinguish all the flaming arrows of the evil one. I put on the helmet of salvation and the sword of the Spirit, which is the Word of God. And most importantly, I will pray in the Spirit all day today. Lord, fight this battle against food for me today. Honor my efforts to develop a healthy relationship with food. I give You total control of my life and of everything I put in my mouth. May I honor You with the choices I make today. Convict me, guide me, and direct me. Amen.

Pause now for a moment in God's Word.

Daily Devotion — Day 16

Read Ephesians 6:10-20. Key verses: Ephesians 6:10-18.

Finally, be strong in the Lord and in his mighty power. Put on the
_____ _____ of _____ so that you can take your
stand against the devil's schemes. For our struggle is not against
flesh and blood, but against the _____, against the authorities, against the powers of this _____ _____ and
against the spiritual forces of _____ in the heavenly realms.
Therefore, put on the _____ armor of _____, so that
when the day of evil comes, you may be able to stand your ground,

91

and after you have done everything, to stand. _____
_____ then, with the _____ of _____ buckled
around your waist, with the _____ of _____ in place,
and with your feet fitted with the _____ that comes from the
_____ of peace. In addition to all this, take up the
_____ of _____, with which you can extinguish all the
flaming _____ of the _____ one. Take
the _____ of _____ and the sword of the
_____, which is the word of _____. And
_____ in the _____ on all occasions with all
kinds of _____ and requests.

These are some of the most powerful verses of Scripture we have. When you face your journey of life each day without putting on the full armor of God, it is like going into war with no weapons. Why face your battles alone? Ask God for help! With His help the victory is yours!

Your spiritual challenge:
Put on your full armor of God daily.

🍎 Food Diary	🙏 Your Prayer

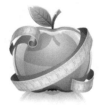

Day 17

The Belt of Truth and Breastplate of Righteousness

Put on the belt of truth. How can you do this? Be truthful with yourself:

- Pray God will reveal areas in your diet you need to work on.

- Accept responsibility for your weight and your eating habits.

- Commit to developing a healthy lifestyle.

Next, put on the breastplate of righteousness. Do this by guarding your heart. Identify those foods closest to your heart: comfort foods, foods you dearly love, foods you crave.

First, look at *comfort foods*. As noted in chapter 2, comfort foods are those foods that soothe you and make you feel warm and content inside: chicken soup when you are sick, hot chocolate with marshmallows on a freezing night, ice cream on a scorching hot day. This category also includes those foods you dearly love: Mama's fried chicken and mashed potatoes, chocolate chip cookies, or homemade strawberry cake.

Remember, God wants you to enjoy food. Food should bring you pleasure. So work your favorite foods and comfort foods into your diet. You can do this by planning ahead. You can decrease your calories throughout the day to save room for food you know you are going to enjoy later. Also, you can cook enough for only one serving of your favorite dish so you won't be tempted to go back for seconds.

To further guard your heart, you will want to eat at the table with the TV off and no distractions. This will help you truly enjoy the food. If you are eating with your family, you can also enjoy the family time. Family mealtime is a very important time of bonding and reconnecting with each other after a day when everyone has been going in different directions.

Finally, let's think about the food you crave. If you totally cut out foods such as chocolate, your favorite desserts, or snacks, you are going to crave them even more. These foods need to be worked into your diet in small amounts and less frequently instead of total eliminating them. Thanks to some ingenious packaging and marketing, you can buy "fun size" chocolate bars or 100 calorie snack packs of many common foods. By eating one or two "fun size" bars or one 100 calorie snack pack, you can enjoy the foods you crave without totally blowing your diet.

Did You Know?

Your local church can provide both support and encouragement. If you have a home church, get active in it. If you don't have one, visit local churches until you find one. Ask a Christian friend to help you. Step out in faith and ask God to help you join the church where He wants you.

Pause now for a moment in God's Word.

Daily Devotion — Day 17

Read Psalm 3:1-8. Key verses: Psalm 3:3-4.

But you are a _____ around me, O Lord; you bestow _____ on me and lift up my head. To the Lord I cry aloud, and he answers me from His holy hill.

Always look to God when you need a shield from temptation.

Small Changes Reap Lasting Rewards

A man reaps what he sows (Galatians 6:7).

Each small change you make builds on the other. Commit to making changes in your eating habits today. Put a check by the changes you are willing to make:

☐ Decrease serving sizes.　　☐ Increase physical activity.

☐ Decrease snacking.　　☐ Decrease intake of fatty foods.

☐ Decrease fat in cooking.　　☐ Decrease intake of sweets.

☐ Keep your food diary.　　☐ Increase vegetables.

☐ Increase water intake.　　☐ Increase fruit intake.

Your spiritual challenge:
Each time you pray before a meal to bless your food, add a prayer for willpower and self-control to keep you from overeating.

Your fitness challenge:
Add an extra ten minutes to your exercise routine today.

The Belt of Truth and Breastplate of Righteousness

Food Diary	Your Prayer

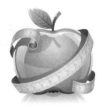

DAY 18

Feet Fitted for Readiness

Are your feet fitted for the readiness, which comes from the gospel of peace? Do you remember the song with the lyrics, "Oh, be careful little feet where you go for the Father is looking down in love, so be careful little feet where you go." Where are places you go that you know are going to tempt you to overeat? Some places are going to really test your will power: an all-you-can-eat buffet, a restaurant that serves extra large servings, or a restaurant that serves all the favorite foods you can't resist. By visiting these places, it may be next to impossible to resist the temptation to overeat; do yourself a favor—don't go there!

Buffets are dangerous. First of all, you pay so much for them, you just have to get your money's worth. Secondly, most of the foods on the buffet are loaded with fat and calories. It is also difficult to tell how the food is prepared. Many times the food is fried then disguised with a sweet and innocent looking sauce to make it not look fried. The vegetables, which should be good for you usually, have tons of calories due to the fat in the seasoning. Beware of buffets.

Stay away from restaurants that are going to test your self-control. Most restaurants have healthy choices on their menus. If you can go to your favorite restaurant and order from the healthy side of the menu, then go and enjoy. However, if you can't resist the foods loaded with fat and calories, then you better eat somewhere else until you have had more practice at recognizing what a healthy plate looks like for you.

Another test of willpower is the grocery store. Don't go to the grocery store feeling hungry or without a list. Have you ever noticed when you shop hungry, you tend to grab everything in sight and end up spending more than you intended? In addition, you will probably end up with more snacks and junk food than you wanted to buy.

Failure to plan is planning to fail. Plan ahead, take time to eat a healthy snack and make out a detailed grocery list before you go to the store. Plan your list around the design of the store so you don't waste time walking from one end of the store to the other searching for items on your list. For example, group all canned foods together, dry goods together, dairy products in another section, and so on.

The longer you stay in the store, the more likely you are to impulse buy. You will have more peace about your diet if you guard your feet so you have control of the foods and temptations to which you are being exposed.

Pause now for a moment in God's Word.

Daily Devotion — Day 18

Read Luke 6:20-26. Key verse: Luke 6:23.

"Rejoice in that day and _____ for joy, because great is your reward in heaven. For that is how their _____ treated the _____."

Jesus tells you to leap for joy when you are hungry: "Blessed are you who hunger now, for you will be satisfied." You are to rejoice and thank God for everything. Romans 8:28 says,

And we know that in all things God works for the good of those who love him, who have been called according to his purpose.

God works in all things for your good. This does not mean all that happens to you is good. Evil is prevalent in our fallen world. However, what it does mean is God is able to turn every circumstance around for your long-term good. This promise is to all people who have accepted Jesus Christ as their Lord and Savior.

This means God wants you to praise Him for the good and the bad happening in your life. God even wants you to praise Him and be joyful in your struggle with your weight. God inhabits your praises. When you praise Him, it releases His power to work in your life in a mighty way. By praising God for your struggles—even your struggle with your weight—it will allow Him to use them for His glory. So look up and praise Him today!

Your nutrition challenge:
Drink eight glasses of water every day.

Food Diary	Your Prayer

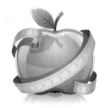

DAY 19

Take Up Your Shield of Faith

Put a shield around your eating habits. You can do this by keeping tempting foods out of sight. You know the old saying, "out of sight, out of mind." Sometimes it helps to get the tempting foods completely out of the house or store them in an inconvenient location. Chocolate, cookies, and other sweets can be stored in the freezer so that you have to plan to eat them.

Do you have a tendency to graze at parties? Counteract the temptation by avoiding going there when you are hungry. Drink a half-cup of juice or a glass of water before the party. If you are really hungry, you may need to eat some raw vegetables, a piece of fruit, or a few crackers before you leave in order to curb your appetite. Plan ahead and decrease your calories at several meals prior to the event. If you must graze, do so on the vegetables and fruits rather than the chips and dips. If you think your host will not have any healthy choices, offer to bring something. If there are several high calorie dishes at the party, pick the one you like the most, eat a moderate amount, and leave the rest for the other guests.

Menu planning can also be a very helpful tool to keep you eating healthy. Plan your menus before you go to the grocery store and buy only the specific foods you need to prepare the planned meals on the menu. Organizing your shopping can help you shop on a budget and ensure you obtain all the items you need for your menu. Look for the low fat, low calorie, and light versions of the foods you normally buy. Let me warn you, when you start cooking more of your meals at home, the cost of your grocery bill may increase. However, the cost of eating away from home should decrease to balance it out.

Following a planned menu should help prevent you from turning to high calorie, quick meals when you are busy during the week. When planning your menus:

- Start with your entrée.
- Add a green, yellow, or orange vegetable, a starch (bread if desired), and a fruit or salad. Always have plenty of color and variety in your menu.

Start a menu and recipe file to keep on hand for recycling. Also keep healthy frozen meals around for emergencies. Plan your menus around your family activities like ball games and school activities, and around your family's favorites and special needs. Develop a daily system such as:

- Grandma's on Sunday
- Pasta on Monday
- Crock-Pot on Tuesday
- Breakfast food on Wednesday
- Casserole on Thursday
- Eat out on Friday
- Grill out on Saturday

RECIPE CORNER
Grape Salad

2 pounds seedless green grapes
2 pounds seedless red grapes
1 (8oz) package of low-fat cream cheese
8 oz light sour cream
1/2 cup sugar substitute
1 tsp. vanilla extract
4 oz chopped pecans
2 Tbsp. brown sugar

Wash and dry grapes. In a large bowl, mix together cream cheese, sour cream, sugar substitute, and vanilla. Add grapes and mix until evenly incorporated. Sprinkle with brown sugar and pecans. Mix again and refrigerate until serving.

Pause now for a moment in God's Word.

Daily Devotion — Day 19

Read Hebrews 12:1-12. Key verse: Hebrews 12:2.

Let us fix our eyes on _____, the author and perfecter of our faith, who for the _____ set before Him endured the cross, scorning its shame, and sat down at the right hand of the throne of God.

Being a Christian is hard work. It requires you give up anything in your life that might be endangering your relationship with God, so you can run with endurance and use the power of the Holy Spirit to help you through your struggles—even your struggle with weight. To have victory in Jesus, you must keep your eyes on Him and away from the enemy. You will stumble if you focus on yourself and your circumstances instead of on the Master.

Your nutrition challenge:
Plan your menu for the week.

Your fitness challenge:
Figure out an exercise that you enjoy
and work it into life at least five days per week.

Live victorious in Jesus today!

🍎 Food Diary	🙏 Your Prayer

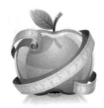

DAY 20

Become a Food Detective

By substituting other items for high calorie foods, it's easy to have a satisfying menu with much lower total fat content and calories.

Original menu example:
fried chicken
macaroni and cheese
purple hull peas
cornbread
sweet tea
TOTAL: 32 grams of fat and 928 calories

Alternate menu with substitutions:
fried chicken	keeping this
corn on the cob	(substituting this for the macaroni and cheese)
green beans	(substituting this for the purple hull peas)
roll	(substituting this for the cornbread)
unsweetened tea	(substituting this for the sweet tea)

TOTAL: 18 grams of fat and 466 calories

Another alternate menu with substitutions:
grilled chicken	(substituting this for the fried chicken)
macaroni and cheese	keeping this
green beans	(substituting this for the purple hull peas)
roll	(substituting this for the cornbread)
unsweetened tea	(substituting this for the sweet tea)

TOTAL: 13.5 grams of fat and 521 calories

> By simply changing the combination of foods but keeping at least one of the foods you love, you can greatly lower your fat and calories.

Compare:

3.5 oz fried chicken	16 grams fat	253 calories
3.5 oz grilled chicken with skin	11 grams fat	222 calories
3.5 oz grilled chicken without skin	4.5 grams fat	173 calories

Compare:

1 slice cornbread	7 grams fat	198 calories
1 roll	1 gram fat	75 calories

Compare:

sweet tea	0 grams fat	110 calories
unsweetened tea	0 grams fat	1 calorie

Compare:

1/2 cup purple hull peas	1 gram fat	112 calories
1/2 cup green beans	0 grams fat	17 calories

Compare:

3/4 cup instant macaroni and cheese	8 grams fat	255 calories
1 small corn on the cob	1 gram fat	120 calories

Did you know not all vegetables were created equally? Starchy vegetables have 80 calories per serving compared to brightly colored vegetables, which have 25 calories per serving. Many of your garden vegetables may actually contribute a lot of extra carbohydrates and calories to your diet when eaten in large amounts. If you are a diabetic, the extra carbohydrates from starchy vegetables may be making it hard to control your blood sugar.

Starchy vegetables are good for you and have their place in a healthy diet when eaten in moderation. Make an effort to only have one starchy vegetable along with one regular vegetable at a meal it will help you lower the calories in your meal.

Starches Versus Vegetables

STARCHES are usually white and dry on the inside.
examples: potatoes, peas, dried beans, and lima beans
80 calories per serving

VEGETABLES are usually juicy and the same color on the inside
as they are on the outside.
examples: green beans, tomatoes, broccoli, and cabbage
25 calories per serving

TOTALLY HEALTHY SUBSTITUTIONS

Instead of:	Have:
fried chicken	grilled chicken
macaroni and cheese	corn on the cob
purple hull peas	green beans
cornbread	roll
sweet tea	unsweetened tea
32 grams Fat	**6.5 grams Fat**
928 Calories	**386 Calories**

As you see from the above example, the menu with substitutions, while still
very tasty, gives you less than half the amount of calories and only 1/6 the
amount of fat! That's quite a difference.

> *Small sacrifices can help save calories*
> *and lead to a lifetime of wellness*
> *while you still eat the food you love.*

Let's compare another meal to help you limit the number of high calorie foods at each meal

Orig. Menu:	Substitute 1:	Substitute 2:
fried fish	fried fish	spicy baked fish
French fries	baked French fries	baked French fries
hush puppies	hush puppies	corn bread
potato salad	cole slaw w/ lt. mayo	turnip greens
regular soda	diet soda	diet soda
47 grams Fat	**31 grams Fat**	**17 grams Fat**
1070 Calories	**700 Calories**	**483 Calories**

Did You Know?

Small groups can be a valuable key to your success. Get a group of friends together that will come along beside you and hold you accountable. Have weekly meetings with Bible study. Weigh in each week and discuss things that are working or not working. Share healthy recipes.

RECIPE CORNER
Light Green Bean Casserole

¾ cup skim milk
1/8 tsp. pepper
1 can 98% fat free cream of mushroom soup
2 cans cut green beans, drained (frozen may also be used)
1 1/3 cup French fried onions

In 1½ quart casserole dish, mix all ingredients except 2/3 cup French onions. Bake 30 minutes at 350° or until hot; stir. Top with 2/3 cup French onions. Bake 5 minutes or until onions are golden.

Pause now for a moment in God's Word.

Daily Devotion — Day 20

Read Ephesians 5:8-14. Key Verse: Ephesians 5:8.

For you were once _____, but now you are _____ in the Lord. Live as children of light.

Have you ever tried to walk around in the dark? In a familiar place you might do fine, but in an unfamiliar one you may end up getting hurt. Think how lost you would feel in a pitch-black room by yourself. You may end up having to crawl to find your way out. If only you had the light from one small candle.

That's the way a person's life is without the light of Christ. Without Christ, you will end up losing your way until you fall on your knees and ask the light of Christ to fill and guide you. Like the light which one candle can give off in a dark room, Christ's light in your life will shine so brightly that you will always be able to find your way. Don't let sin snuff out the light of Christ in your life.

Your nutrition challenge:
Eat a red, yellow or orange vegetable today.

Your fitness challenge:
Walk a mile today.

Live as children of the light!

🍎 **Food Diary**	🙏 **Your Prayer**

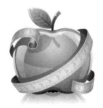

Day 21

The Helmet of Salvation

Put on your helmet of salvation by changing your thought process. Have you ever noticed when you crave a certain food that food is all you can think about until you get it? You need to break this cycle by training yourself to think about something else. You might pray for friends or family or change your activity to help you change your focus.

The devil loves to play mind games with you. He loves to help you beat yourself up, make you feel really bad about yourself, and tempt you with all the foods that are preventing you from losing weight. However, the Scriptures tell us we are children of God, inheritors of the King. Claim that inheritance and your worth. Don't let the devil make you feel like a failure. Don't allow him to put stumbling blocks in your way. His stumbling blocks cause you to keep you focused inward on your own desires rather than upward on Jesus Christ. Ask God to turn those stumbling blocks into building blocks

The Sword of the Spirit, the Word of God

Look up Romans 8:26 and fill in the blanks.
. . . the _____ helps us in our weakness. We do not know what we ought to pray for, but the Spirit himself _____ for us with groans that words cannot express.

Now turn to 2 Corinthians 12:9-10. Paul writes:

But he said to me, "My grace is _____ for you, for my power is made perfect in weakness." Therefore I will boast all the more gladly about my weaknesses, so that Christ's power may rest on me. That is why, for Christ's sake, I delight in weaknesses, in insults, in hardships, in persecutions, in difficulties. For when I am weak, then I am strong.

God's grace is sufficient for all. Allow God's power to be made perfect in your weaknesses with food. Find Scriptures that apply to your individual struggles and claim them every day. God's Word is powerful, especially when you use it in your prayers.

If you were a soldier getting ready to go to war, how would you prepare for your battle? Would you go to the front lines dressed in a pair of jeans, T-shirt, and cap? Or would you put on as much armor and carry as many weapons as you possibly could? Wouldn't you want to be covered from head to toe with armor?

When you start each day without prayer and without covering yourself with the full armor of God, it is like going to war naked. You are leaving yourself open to Satan's attacks. Just as the military has to prepare for battle, we have to prepare for our battle against Satan daily by putting on the full armor of God.

RECIPE CORNER

Low Fat Hot Fries

4-6 potatoes
nonfat butter flavored cooking spray
Creole or Cajun seasoning (to taste)
lemon pepper (to taste)
paprika & pepper (to taste)

Preheat oven to 350°. Peel and cut potatoes into lengthwise wedges. Spray cookie sheet with cooking spray. Place potatoes on top of cookie sheet and spray potatoes with cooking spray. Sprinkle with seasonings. Bake for 45-50 minutes or until potatoes are browned. Turn potatoes occasionally with a spatula.

Pause now for a moment in God's Word.

Daily Devotion — Day 21

Read 2 Corinthians 10:12-18. Key Verse: 2 Corinthians 10:18.

For it is not the one who _____ himself who is approved, but the one whom the _____ commends.

Do you ever find you want to compare yourself to others? I wish I was thin like she is or tall like he is. I wish I was prettier or not so shy. If you think about it, you never measure up, do you? Stop and consider this: God does not ask you to be like someone else. He has given each person unique looks, talents, and gifts to be used in His kingdom. God is the only One from whom you need to seek approval. Forget about what others are doing and ask, "How does my life compare to Jesus Christ?" Seek the approval of God rather the approval of people; when you receive praise you can give God all the credit.

Your spiritual challenge:
Turn to God when you are
tempted to turn to food!

Your nutrition challenge:
Use a smaller plate and fill
at least half the plate with vegetables.

🍎 Food Diary	🙏 Your Prayer

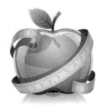

DAY 22

Prayer

The last, but certainly not least, way to put on the full armor of God is through prayer.

And pray in the Spirit on all occasions with all kinds of prayers and requests (Ephesians 6:18).

As Christians, we possess one of the most powerful gifts God could give us—the ability to talk to Him at any time of the day or night. Use that tool to your advantage. If you are unsure how to pray, buy a book on prayer or one that contains prewritten prayers. Prayer works. My hands are living proof of the power of prayer.

In 2004 I faced quite a battle with my health. You could say my body started attacking itself. What started out as a few muscle aches and pains turned into a major attack on my body. My hands and then my feet started swelling. I had no energy and was exhausted all the time.

After a series of tests, the only diagnosis my doctor could provide was hypothyroidism, a fairly simple problem that just required some medicine and everything was supposed return to normal within about six weeks.

During that time, the symptoms grew progressively worse. It was no accident God put a book in my hands about praise and prayer right before these problems began. The book taught me to praise God through all circumstances. I was able to face my illness with praise and with the calm assurance that God was in control.

By the time I returned to my doctor, the tissues in my hands were so inflamed and irritated I had completely lost my range of motion. A minor bump or tug sent pain all the way up my arms. What scared me was my thyroid level was under control; it was evident that something else was very wrong.

My doctor suspected rheumatoid arthritis and referred me to a rheumatologist. That was scary, especially since I was working with an elderly lady who was terribly crippled from rheumatoid arthritis, and our hands had been looking very much alike. I knew firsthand how crippling the disease could be.

Each step of the way I continued to cry out to my Lord and Savior. I think the hardest part about that time was that I knew something was terribly wrong, but I did not know what it was. My husband was out of town the night I returned home from the doctor's visit. Thank goodness for my three boys—the oldest one met me at the car and allowed me to fall into his arms, sobbing. Sometimes you just have to have a meltdown.

I clung to God as our great physician. I went to the rheumatologist; she eventually labeled me with a form of arthritis, which causes hardening of the tissues and skin. It is a very nasty disease with no cure. She diagnosed me purely on symptoms since all my blood tests were still normal. She told me sometimes it takes up to five years for these test to become positive. We couldn't wait that long. She started me on a steroid, and I began giving myself weekly injections.

With the help of medicines, the swelling went down and the pain subsided somewhat. However, I was left with hardening tissues in my hands and arms, which caused carpal tunnel syndrome and limitations on my range of motion and flexibility. I could not make a fist or straighten my hands—they were crippled.

I was referred to a hand specialist, and in January of 2005 I had surgery on my hands to relieve the carpal tunnel syndrome. They also did a biopsy of the thickened skin to see exactly what was happening. The biopsies showed I did have something going on with my tissues but could not positively diagnose or rule out any specific disease.

Prayer and praise became a very important part of my life during that time. Every morning while walking, I would raise my hands and praise God for them. I would drive down the road singing the praise song about taking the shackles off my feet and the chains off my hands, so I could dance and praise Him.

Our God is a faithful God. He will answer our prayers, but He also expects us to do our part. It is like asking God to help you with your diet. You can't just pray, "God, help me to lose weight" but keep eating like you're eating and expect the weight to disappear. You need to ask Him for His help. Praise Him for giving you supernatural self-control. Then you do your part by making changes in your diet and increasing your exercise.

Doing my part on this journey meant some very painful hours of physical therapy. I was referred to a physical therapy center that specialized in hands. They taught my husband and me how to wax and stretch my hands three to four nights a week at home. The therapy was very painful but not nearly as painful as the crazy braces they had me wear. The first pair looked like flippers, and they were to be worn at night while I slept. They were designed to keep my hands stretched out while I slept so my hands would not curl.

It seemed like a pretty good plan, and the braces looked pretty harmless. I thought, *No problem. I will just put them on when I go to bed, get a good night's sleep, and take them off in the morning.* Wrong. The first night I wore them, I woke up every thirty minutes in extraordinary pain. The tissues in my hands were hard and stiff, making them draw in and curl up. So putting something on them that made them stretch out hurt really badly. It would be like taking your fingers and stretching them as far back as they will go and holding them there for hours.

I ended up moving to the couch, wearing a brace on one hand at a time, and changing them off and on all night. This went on for several weeks. Every time I went back to the physical therapist, they would take measurements to see if I had made any improvements.

My progress was slow. I finally started having a difficult time sleeping in the braces. I would put them on when I went to bed, and then my hands would wait until I was asleep and say, "Okay, she's asleep—take them off." And I would wake up with them off every morning.

The therapists then decided to make some more dramatic braces I could wear during the day—four hours on each hand. I called them my scissor hands. They were designed to put my fingers in traction. You've probably seen a person with a broken leg or arm who has the limb hanging in the air in traction. That is the way these braces worked. They were very awkward and painful to wear. With metal rods sticking out everywhere, they looked wild! I would have to take my fingers out of these about every thirty minutes to rest them. This regimen proved very painful.

This went on about four to five months. About a month or so into the physical therapy, I went to a women's meeting. God had laid it on the heart of the woman who was speaking to go around the room and pray over each one of us. I knew the woman but had not seen her in the past year. She had no idea about the struggles I was enduring.

When she prayed over me, she said she closed her eyes and saw Jesus standing behind me stretching my arms and hands out long and straight, and Satan trying to pull them in. Her prayer was God would stretch out my hands to increase my ministry. Her prayer gave me hope and determination to persevere.

Life continued. Then came a sad day about four to five months into physical therapy. When I went for a follow-up with the hand doctor, he told me my hands would never get any better, that once the tissues hardened like mine had done, it was irreversible. The physical therapist told me since I had shown very little improvement over the last couple of months, I should discontinue my appointments. However, if I did not continue to wear the braces or sleep in the splints, my hands would start curling again and would get worse. She very coldly told me there was no hope of improvement. I just needed to work on maintaining.

I quit wearing the scissor braces shortly after that because they were too painful to wear if they were not helping. I tried to sleep in the splints, but my hands would pull them off after I fell sleep no matter how secure I made them.

I gave up on the braces, but I did not give up on God. Many prayers were offered on my behalf at that time. God was faithful. The most amazing thing starting happening—not overnight, but gradually my hands began to improve. The hardened tissues began softening, the swelling in the joints went down, and in October 2005, I took my last injection of medicine. I discontinued all medicine except for the thyroid pills.

My fingers—which had increased by two ring sizes—are now normal. Their range of motion has returned, and I can straighten my fingers out and make a fist without any pain or problems. They have straightened out against all medical odds. So you see, I am living proof prayer works.

Looking back, I believe when the woman prayed over me that night, she was not only praying for my healing but also for this ministry. She prayed God would stretch out my hands and increase my ministry so it reaches far and wide. I did not have a ministry at the time, but God laid this program on my heart soon afterwards. I believe He took me through the valley to prepare me to do His work.

He healed my hands—not to make me more comfortable, not because I'm special, but for one reason and one reason only—to bring Him glory, honor, and praise. He healed me so He can be glorified through me.

Likewise He is going to help you lose weight, not so you can get the glory, or not so *The 40 Day Diet Makeover* can be glorified. This book is the vehicle He is going to use to get to you. God is going to help you lose weight so He can be glorified through you. When someone says to you, "Man, you look great. You've lost a lot of weight. How did you do it?" I want to respond, "I did it by the grace of God through the help of *The 40 Day Diet Makeover.*" It is not about me; it is not about you; it is all about Him.

Our job is to believe in His power. Our lack of faith is what sometimes inhibits God's work in our lives. So pray about this diet and all the other crazy things going on in your life, then praise God that He is in control and helping you fight whatever battle you might face.

The battle to get control of your eating habits and have a healthier life style does not need to be yours alone. Allow God to fight the battles for you by putting on the full armor of God daily.

Pause now for a moment in God's Word.

Daily Devotion — Day 22

Read Luke 10:17-24. Key Verse: Luke 10:19.

Have you analyzed your prayer life lately? How does prayer fit into your life? How do you use prayer on a daily basis?

Prayer is a very powerful tool. In Luke 10:19, God says, "I have given you authority to trample on snakes and scorpions and to overcome all the power of the enemy; nothing will harm you." How do you obtain this authority? Through prayer.

With prayer you can protect yourself from the attacks of the evil one. The Bible says you are to pray without ceasing. So how do you do this? You can't stay on your knees 24/7, but you can start each day with a devotion and prayer. Invite God, through the Holy Spirit, to be a part of your day and talk to Him throughout the day wherever you are.

Prayer gives us a perpetual line of open communication with God. Through prayer you will truly get in tune with God and let Him be the focus of your life. You can do so much more with Him than you could ever do by yourself.

Your fitness challenge:
Add ten minutes of activity
to your lifestyle every day this week.

🍎 **Food Diary**	🙏 **Your Prayer**

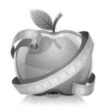

Day 23

Detection or Deception?

Are you a slave to food and your diet? Do you find yourself using food for comfort, stress release, or reward?

Look up 2 Corinthians 11:14-15 and fill in the blanks.

. . . for Satan himself _____ as an angel of light. It is not surprising then, if his servants masquerade as servants of righteousness.

Look up 2 Peter 2:18-19 and fill in the blanks.

For they mouth empty, boastful words and, by appealing to the lustful desires of _____ human nature, they entice people who are just escaping from those who live in error. They promise them freedom, while they themselves are slaves of depravity—for a man is a slave to whatever has mastered him.

Don't allow Satan to make you a slave to food. Food is *deceptive*. Look up Proverbs 23:1-3 and fill in the blanks.

When you sit to dine with a ruler, note well what is before you, and put a _____ to your _____ if you are given to gluttony. Do not crave his delicacies for that food is deceptive.

The devil uses food to entice you by telling you food will comfort you, will help you relax, or that you deserve a reward. For example, "You deserve that hot fudge sundae. After all, you've had a really hard week."

Food is *addictive*. Sometimes, once you start eating, you can't quit. It's hard to eat just one. Abusing your body by overeating is just as much a sin as abusing your body with alcohol or drugs.

Overeating Needs To Stop

As indicated in chapter 1, you need to rebirth your body's natural instincts. Be aware of when you are hungry, when you are full, and the amount of food you should eat at one time.

Build hedges around your eating habits. Those hedges will help you eat less automatically. You can do such things as:

- *Use smaller plates.* Some of us think we have to eat an entire plate of food at every meal. If you use a smaller plate, you can decrease your serving sizes and still eat a plate of food. It tricks you into eating less.

- *Drink water or juice before meals.* Drink sixteen ounces of water or a half-cup of juice or eat a piece of fruit before meals. When you feel extremely hungry, you tend to overeat. Drinking water or juice or eating fruit will put something in your stomach so you won't be as hungry when you eat your meal.

- *Don't skip meals.* As a general rule, people who skip meals consume more calories per day than people who eat three meals and one to two snacks per day. Eating small amounts throughout the day stimulates metabolism.

- *Chew your food slowly.* Since your brain takes twenty minutes to tell your stomach you are full, taking your time when you are eating will help you enjoy every bite and give you time to feel full. Eat slowly. If you are starting to feel the least bit full, stop eating even if you still have food on your plate that will go to waste. It's better to waste than to wear.

- *Don't eat every meal as if it is your last meal.* Unless you live in a country where food is unavailable, I feel certain you will be able to eat again. So don't eat all the calories you need in one day at one meal.

- *Portion out your snacks.* Eating from a bag is dangerous, unless you are eating a pre-portioned snack or a 100 calorie snack pack. Even healthy snacks can add unwanted calories to your diet without portion control. Therefore, weigh or measure your snacks into sandwich or snack bags. Take them to work, on outings, or have them stored in your cabinet at home. Then, when you walk in the kitchen starving, you will have a snack ready and will not be as tempted to eat the fattening snacks—or overeat healthy snacks and get unwanted calories.

Decrease fat in your diet. Start paying attention to how you are cooking and make a conscious effort to cook your food healthier! Remember there are 3,500 calories in one pound of body fat. Fat has more calories than any other nutrients. Fat has nine calories per gram compared to carbohydrates and protein with only four calories per gram. Therefore, an easy way to cut calories in your diet is to decrease your fat intake. While some fat is good for you, too much fat can pile on extra calories and lead to unwanted health problems.

Pause now for a moment in God's Word.

Daily Devotion — Day 23

Read James 1:1-18. Key Verses: James 1:2-3.

Consider it pure _____, my brothers, whenever you face trials of many kinds, because you know that the _____ of your faith develops _____.

At times, the battle with your weight might seem endless—a constant trial that you must face. Weight management is not something that can be achieved quickly; it takes hard work and perseverance. But by the grace of God, you have VICTORY in Jesus! He will supply you with all you need to persevere and win the battle.

Build hedges around your eating habits by committing to making some of the changes below.

- Use smaller plates.
- Drink 16 oz. of water or 1/2 cup of 100% juice before meals.
- Don't skip meals.
- Chew your food slowly.
- Pre-portion your snacks.
- Don't eat when you are not hungry.
- Decrease your fat intake

Your nutrition challenge:
Commit to making at least
one of these changes each week.

Your fitness challenge:
Increase the intensity of your exercise today.

Detection or Deception?

🍎 Food Diary	🙏 Your Prayer

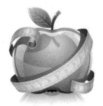

Day 24

Facts You Should Know

Twenty-five to thirty percent of your calories should come from fat. For a 1,800 calorie diet, you only need 50-60 grams of fat daily.

Calculating Fat Grams

Calories per day x 30 percent = fat calories—the maximum number of calories you need from fat per day. Then divide that result by nine since fat has nine calories per gram.

For example:
1500 calories x .30 = 450 calories from fat
450 calories ÷ 9 calories per gram = 50 grams

This means a person consuming 1500 calories per day should eat a total of only 50 grams of fat per day.

Types of Fat

There are three kinds of fat:

• saturated fats
• monounsaturated fats
• polyunsaturated fats

Monounsaturated fats are the best for you because they are easily digested by the body. They are liquid at room temperature. Sources of monounsaturated fat are: olive, peanut and canola oils.

Polyunsaturated fats are also a better fat for your body. They are not as good for you as monounsaturated fats, but they are better for you than saturated fats. They are liquid or soft at room temperature. Sources of polyunsaturated fats are: safflower, sunflower, corn, soybean and cottonseed oils.

Saturated fats are bad fats because saturated and trans fat have a substance called plaque in them which adheres to arterial walls. The greater amount of this kind of fat in your diet, the greater the health risk. Saturated fats are solid at room temperature. and are mainly found in animal products. However, they can be found in some plant sources such as coconut. Saturated fats should make up no more than 10 percent of your calories.

Keep in mind all fats have approximately the same number of calories per serving. The difference is in the way your body handles these fats. Don't fool yourself into thinking it is okay to eat fried food often because you are using a healthier fat. Fried food will still add unwanted calories.

Tablespoon per tablespoon, all fats have 100-120 calories. However, because they are prepared differently, they may vary in calories. Tub margarine is whipped, which causes it to contain more air and water; therefore, it has fewer calories per tablespoon than stick margarine. However, if you melt both of these margarines and remove the water, they would have the same number of calories. The extra water in tub margarine sometimes causes it not to be a good substitute for stick margarine in recipes.

You need to also beware of trans fats. The process of hydrogenation, adding hydrogen to a liquid vegetable oil to make it solid, causes the formation of trans fat. It is highest in stick margarine, snack foods, and baked goods like cookies. Trans fats are also found in commercially fried foods like French fries.

All food labels are required by law to list trans fats, which are like a double whammy to your health. They have not only been accused of raising the bad cholesterol—LDL cholesterol—they also lower the good cholesterol, HDL. Research has shown links to chronic diseases and trans fats.

Some trans fats are found naturally in dairy products and meat. However, the trans fats made by God do not have the same negative effects on our health as the trans fats from hydrogenation by man.

Your nutritional challenge:
Decrease your fat intake.

Pause now for a moment in God's Word.

Daily Devotion — Day 24

Read Galatians 6:7-10. Key Verse: Galatians 6:7-8.

A man reaps what he sows. The one who sows to please his sinful nature, from that nature will reap destruction; the one who sows to please the Spirit, from the Spirit will reap eternal life.

You reap what you sow. However, it is not immediate. It sometimes takes years of poor eating habits and unhealthy lifestyle to cause destruction. It may also take years for the damage to be reversed. Pray for patience because the seeds you sow today will help you reap a healthier tomorrow.

Your nutrition challenge:
Sow healthy seeds
today for a healthier tomorrow.

Your spiritual challenge:
Get up thirty minutes earlier
every day this week for extra devotion and prayer time.

Your fitness challenge:
Put a spring in your step
and make every step count today.

🍎 **Food Diary**	🙏 **Your Prayer**

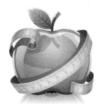

DAY 25

Controlling Your Cholesterol and Fat Levels

Cholesterol is a waxy substance made by the liver and found in the diet. Its job is to transport fat in the body from one place to another—like the body's taxi service for fat. Cholesterol levels should be less than 200; 200-239 is considered borderline high.

You have probably gone to the doctor and heard him talk about your HDL and LDL cholesterol. What was he talking about? To put it in simple terms, I call the HDL cholesterol your "happy cholesterol" because it takes fat from the body to the liver to be used for energy. It gets fat out of your body. Exercise is very helpful in increasing your HDL levels. HDL levels should be high—no less than fifty milligrams per deciliter (1/10 of a liter or 100 milliliters) or fifty milligrams per deciliter for women and no less than forty milligrams per deciliter for men.

I call your LDL your "lousy cholesterol" because it takes fat from the liver and stores it in the tissues. You want these levels to be below 100 mg/dl.

The more calories you get from fat, the greater risk you will be for weight gain, heart attacks, or strokes. If your diet is high in cholesterol and saturated fat, these fats contribute to the development of arterial plaque. As plaque builds up, it sticks to the walls of the arteries. This blocks the pathway for blood to flow, which places stress on your heart.

If plaque completely blocks the flow to the heart, it will cause a heart attack. If plaque completely blocks the flow to the brain, it will cause a stroke. You need to decrease the fat you are eating by decreasing the fat in cooking. You can do this by:

• Cooking with a nonstick skillet.
• Cooking with spray oil instead of butter, shortening, or oil.

- Cooking with low fat or light margarines.
- Substituting applesauce for oil in recipes such as cake mixes, brownies, or muffin mixes. If the recipe calls for a half-cup of oil, you can use half-cup of applesauce instead. In dark foods—brownies or chocolate cake—you can substitute baby food prunes or applesauce in place of the oil. This is an easy way to decrease the fat without altering the taste.
- Using the low fat, light, or fat free versions of sour cream, nondairy whipped topping, or salad dressing.
- Use low fat cheese.

The table below shows some substitutes with a comparison of fats and calories to their counterparts.

Small Substitutions = Big Calorie and Fat Savings

Sour Cream	1 tablespoon	26 calories	2.5 gm fat
	1 cup	416 calories	40 gm fat
Light Sour Cream	1 tablespoon	18 calories	0.7 gm fat
	1 cup	288 calories	11 gm fat
Butter	1 tablespoon	102 calories	12 gm fat
Light Margarine	1 tablespoon	70 calories	7 gm fat
Whole Milk	1 cup	150 calories	8 gm fat
Skim Milk	1 cup	86 calories	0.4 gm fat
Bologna	1 ounce	90 calories	8 gm fat
Turkey Bologna	1 ounce	60 calories	4.5 gm fat
Smoked Ham	1 ounce	22 calories	1 gm fat
Soft Drink	20 ounces	258 calories	0 gm fat
Diet Soft Drink	20 ounces	0 calories	0 gm fat

In most recipes you can substitute low fat, fat free, or sugar free without changing the quality of the recipe. The light banana pudding recipe on the next page is an example.

Light Banana Pudding

1 box sugar free vanilla pudding mix
2-3 cups skim milk
12 oz. light nondairy whipped topping
Vanilla wafers
6 bananas
Mix pudding with milk according to directions. Fold in the whipped topping. Layer pudding mixture with a few vanilla wafers and sliced bananas.

The following chicken quesadilla recipe shows how to calculate the number of calories per serving. Try calculating the calories per serving in your own recipes at home.

Chicken Quesadillas

Ingredients	Amount	Calories	Fat
Boneless chicken breast	4	420	12 grams
Taco seasoning	1 package	trace amt.	trace amt.
Diced tomatoes	1 can	68	0 grams
6-in flour tortilla	8	640	8 grams
Low fat mozzarella cheese	1 cup	576	36 grams
Low fat cheddar cheese	1/2 cup	360	12 grams
Low fat sour cream	1/2 cup	144	5.6 grams
Salsa	1/2 cup	67	0 grams
Water	1/2 cup	0	0 grams
Cooking spray		0	0 grams
TOTAL		2,275	73.6 grams

2,275 calories ÷ 8 servings/recipe = **284 calories/serving**
74 grams fat ÷ 8 servings/recipe = **9 grams fat/serving**

Directions: Cook chicken in a crock pot or slow oven with taco seasoning and tomatoes for 6-8 hours. Take chicken out and cut or shred into small pieces. On half of a flour tortilla, layer chicken and cheese; fold other half over as though you were making an omelet. Place in hot skillet or on griddle that has been sprayed with cooking oil. Cook until brown on both sides. Serve with sour cream and salsa.

Meats contribute a great deal of fat to your diet, especially if they are not cooked in a healthy way. Below are some tips to help in this area.

- Trim off all the visible fat.
- Twice boil meats for casseroles and soups. Boil the meat, pour off the water, then boil it again before using it in your soup or casserole.
- Boil ahead of time and refrigerate. Then scrape the fat off before using it in the recipe.
- Bake, boil, broil, or grill your meats instead of frying them.
- Stir-fry in a nonstick skillet or with one to two teaspoons of olive oil.
- Remove as much fat from your food after cooking as possible. To do this, drain off fat after cooking, blot with a paper towel, strain in a colander, and rinse with hot water.

Pause now for a moment in God's Word.

Daily Devotion — Day 25
Read Jonah 2:1-10. Key Verse: Jonah 2:2.

"In my _____ I called to the Lord, and He answered me. From the _____ of the grave I called for help, and you _____ to my cry."

Are you running from God? If you are a Christian, you have a calling in your life. It may be something simple like showing compassion to a friend, helping the needy, sending cards to people, being a prayer warrior, or singing in the church choir. It may be something bigger like teaching Sunday school, leading a Bible study, getting involved in missions, being a leader in your church, or being in ministry. Sometimes it is hard for us to do what God is calling us to do because of self. Pray God will hide you behind His cross so He can use you for His glory. Step out in faith and let God use you to reach His people one person at a time.

Your spiritual challenge:

Step out in faith to do what God is calling you to do so His power can be released to work in your life.

🍎 **Food Diary**	🙏 **Your Prayer**

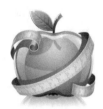

Day 26

Guilt Free Eating Out

You can avoid unwanted fat and calories when eating out. Choose foods that are prepared in a low fat way.

- Ask the waiter to hold the cheese and the mayonnaise. In general, adding a slice of cheese or one tablespoon of mayonnaise to a burger adds about ten grams of fat. Therefore, hold the cheese and the mayonnaise. Add mustard, ketchup, and pickles instead.

- Ask for butter, sour cream, and dressing on the side so you can control how much of it you use.

- Order smaller servings—child size or appetizers.

- Ask for a to-go box for leftovers so you will not feel you are wasting your food or feel you have to eat the entire portion.

Choose meals wisely

Instead of:	Choose:
chicken salad sandwich on white bread with lettuce and tomato	turkey sandwich on whole wheat bread with mozzarella cheese, lettuce, tomatoes, and mustard.
potato chips	pretzels
pickle spear (OK, no change)	pickle spear
1 cup fruit punch	1 cup skim milk
579 calories and 26 grams fat	**447 calories and 5 grams fat**

Instead of:	Choose:
8 ounce steak	6 ounce grilled chicken breast
French fries	baked potato with sour cream
1 roll	steamed vegetables
12 ounce regular soda	12 ounce diet soda
1,160 calories and 41 grams fat	**724 calories and 13 grams fat**

Read Philippians 3:18-20 and fill in the blanks.

For, as I have often told you before and now say again even with tears, many live as _____ of the cross of Christ. Their destiny is _____, their god is their stomach, and their glory is in their shame. Their mind is on earthy things. But our _____ is in heaven. And we eagerly await a Savior from there, the Lord Jesus Christ, who, by the power that enables Him to bring everything under His control, will transform our lowly bodies so that they will be like His glorious body.

Continuing with the next verse, Philippians 4:1.

Therefore, my brothers, you whom I love and long for, my joy and crown, that is how you should stand firm in the Lord, dear friends!

So how are you going to conquer your battle with the bulge? By standing firm in the Lord!

I can do everything through him who gives me strength (Philippians 4:13).

Like Paul in Philippians 4:11, we need to learn to be content with less! *"...for I have learned to be content whatever the circumstances."*

Daily Devotion — Day 26

Read Mark 10:27-31. Key Verse: Mark 10:27.

Jesus looked at them and said, "With man this is impossible, but not with God; all things are possible with God."

Sometimes it seems as if it is impossible to lose even one pound, much less five or ten more pounds. Alone, it may be impossible. However, with God all things are possible. Put your trust in God today and allow Him to make your impossible, possible.

Your spiritual challenge:
Practice trusting God with every aspect of your life today.

Your fitness challenge:
Spend more time moving around and being active than sitting today.

With Christ you can do all things.
Even the impossible becomes possible!

🍎 Food Diary	🙏 Your Prayer

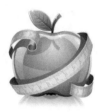

DAY 27

Bring Something Healthy

Jenny came to the women's Bible study so excited. She said to her friends,

I just have to tell you about my new diet. It is so easy. I just know you will want to try it. I have already lost five pounds in five days. Yep, a pound a day. That's the promise. This is how it works.

All you have to do is wear this band on your ear with these little wires sticking out of it. The band sends rays to the sun; the rays go to your stomach, mix around, and come out through your eyes to help you see food in a whole new light. It makes you not want to eat, because the food does not look or smell good to you. It works, it really does and it only costs two hundred dollars.

Jenny said she was taking orders for them. Would you buy one? It sounds too good to be true, doesn't it? Have you ever been on a diet? If you have, you have probably figured out by now that most diets do not work for long-term weight loss. They may work while you are on them, but they quickly stop working as soon as you get off them. On-again, off-again diets cause you to end up with some or all of the weight being regained. Most diets make you feel very trapped, stressed, out of control, or very restricted. Avoid the temptation to jump on the fad diet bandwagon. Falling off of it is too easy.

Pause now for a moment in God's Word.

Daily Devotion — Day 27

Read Ephesians 4:14-16. Key Verse: Ephesians 4:16.

From him the whole body, joined and held together by every
_____ _____, grows and builds itself up
in _____, as each part does its _____.

Your body is a gift from God, put together to work like a fine-tuned machine. Take care of this gift, treasure and honor it.

Imagine you have been on this program for four weeks, and you have started making changes in your eating habits, started exercising, and have even lost ten pounds. Then you and your friends plan a going away party for a friend at work. There will be plenty of food loaded with fat and calories. Someone volunteered to bring a cake, another chips and dip, another punch, another nuts, and still another is bringing hot wings. What should you volunteer to bring?

- ☐ cheese dip and chips
- ☐ ice cream to go with the cake
- ☐ vegetable and fruit tray with low fat dip
- ☐ diet drink

If you bring something healthy to eat and drink, you will be able to eat more. What should you do if your friends want to eat Mexican for lunch two hours before the party?

- ☐ Go eat with them and order your favorite meal.
- ☐ Talk them into waiting until another day.
- ☐ Go with them and order a small salad, no chips.

Save calories by eating a light breakfast and lunch so you can eat some of your favorite food at the party. Thinking out situations like this ahead of time will prepare you for success.

Your spiritual challenge:
Pray daily for the Holy Spirit to guard your
steps at keep you out of Satan's traps.

🍎 Food Diary	🙏 Your Prayer

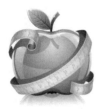

DAY 28

To Diet or Not To Diet

How many of you went to bed at your ideal weight one night and woke up the next morning twenty or more pounds heavier? Most weight and health problems don't start with one single event in your life. Rather, they are from an accumulation of events that happen over years. However, we expect these problems to be corrected with one single diet or pill. Fad diets are usually expensive, very restrictive, and boring. They are a short-term, quick fix approach to a long-term problem.

That's why the devil loves for you to go on a fad diet; he knows you are setting yourself up for failure. Like a yo-yo, your weight will go up and down on fad diets. Dieting can be a vicious cycle. If you get caught in the cycle, you may find yourself dieting very strictly, losing weight, cheating, beating yourself up and feeling terrible (shattering your self-esteem), then buying into another fad diet. Research shows as many as 95 percent of the people who go on a fad diet regain the weight in one to five years.

Fad diets are not the answer!

Contrary to what advertisers say, fad diets are not the answer to your weight problem. Losing weight is difficult, yet that is the promise of all the fad diets: quick and easy. A general rule for fad diets is, if it sounds too good to be true, it probably is. Before you jump on a fad diet bandwagon, ask the following questions:

- Does it promise quick and easy weight loss?
- Does it sound too good to be true?

- Does it promise results without physical activity or a change in lifestyle?
- Does it promote good versus bad food?
- Does it exclude food from a certain food group?
- Is it expensive?
- Does it promote a specific product?
- Is it too structured and not family friendly?

Did you answer yes to any of these questions? They are red flags to look for when evaluating fad diets. Learning about nutrition and the nutrients that make up the food you are eating will help you make more informed decisions about your eating habits. The following recipe makes a great breakfast or can be served for a healthy, great tasting dessert.

RECIPE CORNER
Yogurt Fruit Sundae

2 bananas – cut in half, quartered and sliced
1 apple – peeled and diced
1 can mandarin oranges, drained
1 cup honeydew melon – cut in bite sized pieces (optional)
1 cup cantaloupe – cut in bite sized pieces(optional)
1 cup blueberries, strawberries (cut in half), or raspberries
1) 8 oz. container of berry flavored low fat yogurt
6 tsp. wheat germ or chopped pecans
2 kiwi fruit, peeled and sliced (optional)

In the order listed, place prepared fruit into four stemmed individual crystal dessert dishes. Top each serving with ¼ of the container of yogurt. Top the yogurt with wheat germ or chopped pecans. Place a kiwi slice on top.

Pause now for a moment in God's Word.

Daily Devotion — Day 28

Read Nehemiah 8:9-10. Key Verse: Nehemiah 8:10.

. . . the _____ of the Lord is your strength.

Who is the source of your joy? The *New King James* version of the verse above says, "Do not sorrow, for the joy of the Lord is your strength." If you are trying to find joy from your job, your spouse, your friends, your possessions, or your successfulness at losing weight, you will be sorely disappointed. All you will find is emptiness, discontentment, and hopelessness.

Start today putting Christ first and watch your life turn around. You will discover that He alone is the source of the love, peace, and joy for which you have been searching. Simply being in the presence of God will bring you great joy.

Your nutrition challenge:
Don't eat anything fried this weekend.

Your spiritual challenge:
Strive for true joy in your daily life.

Don't forget to weigh yourself weekly and plot it on the graph in the front of the book.

🍎 **Food Diary**	🙏 **Your Prayer**

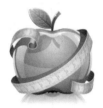

DAY 29

Nutrition 101

Our food is made up of three macronutrients: carbohydrates, fats, and protein. These are needed by our body to supply energy and build tissue. Our food also contains many micronutrients—vitamins and minerals the body uses in much smaller amounts to regulate and control body processes. Our body must also have the vital nutrient, water, which is essential for sustaining all our life processes.

The first macronutrient is *carbohydrates*, the focus of many fad diets. Carbohydrates are your body's main source of energy. In fact, they are your brain's most important source of energy. They were made by God to be used as an immediate source of energy for our body's daily energy expenditure: getting out of bed, walking, cleaning, exercising, and most importantly, thinking.

Carbohydrates can also be stored by the body's muscle tissue in the form of glycogen, the body's main source of energy during exercise. Therefore, when you are limiting carbohydrates, you are restricting a very important source of energy for your body. As with all of these nutrients, too many carbohydrates will add unwanted calories and result in weight gain. However, greatly restricting carbohydrates will result in fatigue, headaches, and other symptoms.

The main sources of carbohydrates are:
- bread
- cereal
- starchy vegetables
- fruits
- milk
- simple sugar

The next macronutrient is *protein*. Protein is important for building and maintaining muscle function. Unless you are a professional body builder, you do not need protein supplements to build muscle. In fact, most Americans eat too much protein, which causes stress on the kidneys. Protein plays a very important role in our body; it helps build muscle and gives your meal substance. Protein will give you a feeling of fullness. Protein will stay with you for a longer period of time than a meal with just fat and carbohydrates. However, keep in mind protein is only needed in small amounts at each meal.

The main sources of protein are:
• meat (beef, fish, pork, poultry)
• eggs
• dried beans and peas
• milk

Fat is our last macronutrient. Fat is important for carrying and storing fat-soluble vitamins. It cushions your organs and regulates body temperature. It is also important for adding flavor to your food. Because it contributes the most calories to your diet, fat is another macronutrient which many fad diets restrict. Since fat plays such a vital role in your body, it should not be totally eliminated. Fat should be limited to small amounts at each meal. As noted earlier, too much fat can be detrimental to your diet and your health.

The sources of fat are:
• oil, margarine, butter
• hidden fats are found in bacon, sausage, processed foods, fried foods

Have you ever heard of Olestra? Olestra—also known by the brand name, Olean—is a fat substitute which has the same characteristics as fat but is not absorbed by the body. Olestra is found mainly in products such as light potato chips. Because it is not absorbed by the body, Olestra may cause diarrhea when eaten in large quantities. As it moves through the body unabsorbed, Olestra pulls out fat-soluble vitamins and nutrients. Therefore, I do not recommend this product to be used in large amounts, especially with children.

All these nutrients play an important role in your body. Do you think God would have given you three nutrients and then said, "But wait, don't eat this one because it is really bad for you"? No, God knows that you need a balanced diet with all three nutrients. It is His plan.

RECIPE CORNER

Vegetable Pizza (a great appetizer to serve at parties)

2 (8 oz) packages refrigerated low fat crescent rolls
2 (8oz) packages low fat cream cheese, softened
1 cup light mayonnaise
1(1 oz) pkg. dry ranch dressing mix
1 cup fresh broccoli, chopped
1 cup chopped tomatoes
1 cup chopped green, red, or yellow bell pepper (optional)
1 cup chopped cauliflower (optional)
1 cup shredded carrots (optional)
1 cup shredded 2 percent cheddar cheese

Preheat oven to 375º. Roll out the crescent roll dough onto a 9 X 13 inch baking sheet and pinch together edges to form the pizza crust.

Bake crust for 12 minutes in the preheated oven. Remove baked crust from oven and let cool 15 minutes without removing it from the baking sheet.

In a small mixing bowl combine cream cheese, mayonnaise, and dry ranch dressing. Spread the mixture over the cooled crust. Arrange broccoli, tomatoes, bell pepper, cauliflower, shredded carrots, and cheddar cheese over the cream cheese layer. Chill for one hour; slice and serve.

Pause now for a moment in God's Word.

Daily Devotion — Day 29

Read Genesis 50:19-21. Key Verse: Genesis 50:20.

"You intended to harm me, but God intended it for _____ to accomplish what is now being done, the _____ of many lives."

Satan wants to take the things that God intended for good and use them for bad. That's not God's plan. He gave you food for your enjoyment, to nourish you and keep you healthy. Allow God to help you modify your diet and lifestyle to reflect the goodness of His plan.

Break the cycle of dieting!

Use common sense when dieting. Remember: if it sounds too good to be true, it probably is! Fad diets are not the answer!

Pop Quiz:

Carbohydrates are your body's main source of: _____

Proteins function to: _____

Fats help us regulate:_____

Fats transport fat soluble: _____

God gave you all three nutrients to work together to nourish your body. No one food or nutrient can nourish your body by itself!

Your spiritual challenge:
Quit looking for a quick fix and ask God to help you make the necessary changes that will lead to a lifetime of weight management.

Your fitness challenge:
Find an exercise plan that works for you and stick to it.

🍎 Food Diary	🙏 Your Prayer

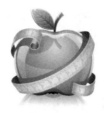

Day 30

Moderation, Not Total Restriction

Look up the first part of 1 Corinthians 12:12 and fill in the blanks.

The body is a unit, though it is made up of many _____; and though all its parts are many, they form _____ body.

Now look at 1 Corinthians 12:18-20.

But in fact God has arranged the parts in the body, every _____ of them, just as He wanted them to be. If they were all _____ part, where would the body be? As it is there are _____ parts, but one body.

Think about it. A nose by itself would be no good without a body, or an eye by itself would be no good without a body. Just as our bodies are made up of many parts, so are the foods God gave us to nourish our bodies. No one food or nutrient can nourish our bodies by itself.

Look up Ephesians 4:16 and fill in the blanks.

From him the whole body, joined and held together by every supporting ligament, grows and builds itself up in _____, as each part does its work.

Beware of fad diets that greatly restrict one of your macronutrients.

While carbohydrates and fats can provide extra, unwanted calories when overeaten, they are an integral part of our diet. The key is moderation. There is a big difference between moderation and total restriction.

Daily Devotion — Day 30

Read Psalm 27:11-14. Key Verse: Psalm 27:14.

Wait for the Lord; be _____ and take heart and wait for the Lord.

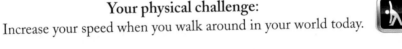

Sometimes you may feel as though you are all alone in your struggles. Your focus is inward on self. The Bible says that in the day of trouble, God will keep you safe in His dwelling (Psalm 27:5). Maybe you need to change your gaze from inward to upward. Wait upon the Lord. Rely on Him through your struggles. Be patient and wait upon the Lord.

Your physical challenge:
Increase your speed when you walk around in your world today.

Your nutrition challenge:
Are you eating your vegetables? Fill half of your plate with a green, yellow, or orange vegetables or salad.

Food Diary	Your Prayer

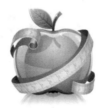

DAY 31

The Wide or the Narrow Road

The broad path to losing weight is easy: a fad diet, a pill, a shot, no real, long-term commitment. Because it is a bandage that relies strictly on self or gimmicks, this approach leads to failure and destruction. As humans we are weak; we can't do it alone. But we can do it with God, relying fully and completely on Him.

The narrow road is challenging. It takes real, lifelong commitment and effort. The rewards do not come quickly but are greater and more lasting.

Look up Proverbs 3:5-6 and fill in the blank.

Trust in the Lord with all your heart and lean not on your own understanding; in all your ways _____ him, and he will make your paths straight.

God never promised us it would be easy; nothing about losing weight and keeping it off is easy. However, He did promise His grace is sufficient for all.

What is grace? Grace is God's unmerited favor. In the words of a child, "It is God treating us a lot better than we deserve to be treated." Jesus is saying, "All you have to do is repent, my child, and ask Me into your life, and I will carry your burdens." Our sinful nature separates us from God. Through grace, it is as if we never sinned.

Accepting Jesus Christ as your Lord and Savior is a beginning, not the end of your walk in faith. Your walk in faith continues throughout your life by God's grace. Through His grace you come to know God and God's will for your life. He has a key to your heart. He is just waiting for an invitation from you. In James 2:17, James said faith without works is dead. We have to put feet to our faith. It needs to be demonstrated in every dimension of our life.

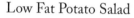

RECIPE CORNER
Low Fat Potato Salad

6 cups red potatoes, unpeeled
½ tsp. garlic powder
1 tsp. lemon juice
1tsp. curry powder
½ cup low fat mayonnaise
½ cup purple or sweet onion, diced (optional)
1 tsp. celery seed
1 tsp. parsley flakes
2 tsp. mustard
1 cup fat free sour cream
salt and black pepper to taste

Boil unpeeled whole potatoes until tender. Cool and cut into desired size. Combine remaining ingredients and add to potatoes. Mix well. May be served immediately or chilled in the refrigerator until ready to serve.

Pause now for a moment in God's Word.

Daily Devotion — Day 31

Look up Matthew 7:13-14 and fill in the blanks. Jesus says:

"Enter through the _____ gate. For wide is the gate and broad is the road that leads to _____, and many enter through it. But _____ is the gate and narrow the road that leads to life, and only a few find it."

Which road will you choose—the wide or the narrow road?

The Narrow Road

hard work
lifelong commitment
permanent changes
success, victory, lasting weight management, and a permanent, healthy lifestyle

The Wide Road

a fad diet
no real commitment
gimmicks
failure and destruction

Your spiritual challenge:
Ask God to help you choose the narrow road today for a healthier tomorrow!

Your fitness challenge:
Exercise is important for helping you maintain a weight loss. Make exercise a part of your daily routine!

Food Diary	Your Prayer

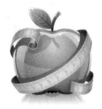

DAY 32

The Seven Characteristics To Develop

The following passage found in 2 Peter 1:5-7 outlines seven character-istics that we, as Christians, should work to develop in our lives:

For this very reason, make every effort to add to your faith good-ness; and to goodness, knowledge; and to knowledge, self-control; and to self-control, perseverance; and to perseverance, godliness; and to godliness, brotherly kindness; and to brotherly kindness, love.

List those seven characteristics below.

1. _____
2. _____
3. _____
4. _____
5 _____
6. _____
7. _____

Specifically, work on developing self-control and perseverance to help you persist through all circumstances of your life, including long-lasting weight management.

Pause now for a moment in God's Word.

Daily Devotion — Day 32

Read Galatians 5:22-25. Key Verses: Galatians 5:22-23.

But the fruit of the Spirit is love, joy, peace, _____, kindness, goodness, faithfulness, gentleness and _____.

Be sensitive to the seeds God is planting in your heart. They are seeds of love, joy, peace, patience, kindness, goodness, faithfulness, gentleness and self-control from the fruit of the Spirit.

Notice I referred to "fruit" and not "fruits." Just as a watermelon is one fruit but has many seeds, so is the fruit of the Spirit one fruit that comes with many seeds God desires to plant in your life. It takes seeds to grow a watermelon as it takes the seeds from the fruit of the Spirit to grow you into a mature Christian.

If you ask Jesus to be Lord and Savior of your life, but have not cultivated the fruit of the Spirit in your life, then you will be like a watermelon with no seeds. The life-giving seeds will be what sustain you when trials come your way. If you cultivate the fruit of the Spirit, those seeds of love, joy, peace, patience, kindness, goodness, faithfulness, gentleness, and self-control will begin to sprout and root deep within. Those seeds will help you be anchored firmly in your faith to withstand the attacks of the evil one.

With the fruit of the Spirit in your life, God can grow you from the inside as he prepares to use you in His kingdom. The seeds from one watermelon can be harvested to produce many sweet, delicious fruits and will continue to multiply. The same is true for you as you work on developing the fruit of the Spirit in your life. Your outer body may deteriorate but your inner self will grow stronger, and you will be able to stand strong against the attacks of Satan. You will be able to influence the lives of many for Christ.

The fruit of the Spirit is developed from a close walk with God by daily meditation on His Word and communication with God in prayer. Jesus says, "I am the true vine and my Father is the gardener" (John 15:1). "If a man remains in me and I in him, he will bear much fruit; apart from me you can do nothing" (John 15:5). The only ways to remain in Him are by reading His Word and through prayer.

Ask God to develop the fruit of the Spirit in your life. Be willing to change as He helps you take off your old self and put on a new self in Christ. Plant His Word deep within your heart so when adversity and trials come your way, you will be able to stand and point others to Christ.

Your spiritual challenge:
Ask God to develop the fruit of the Spirit in your life today.

Your fitness challenge:
Sit less; move more!

🍎 **Food Diary**	🙏 **Your Prayer**

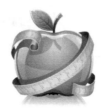

Day 33

Obstacles of Grace

Let's look at grace a little closer. What are your obstacles to grace? What keeps you from accepting the grace God is offering? Is it fear of failure or fear you will have to give up old habits, especially ungodly habits? Maybe it is your fear of losing control. Many times we surrender a portion of our life to Christ but not every aspect of it. Remember, where sin is, God cannot be. You must get sin out of the way to allow God to come in and work in your life.

So how do we overcome these obstacles? First, pray without ceasing. This gives you a perpetual line of open communication with God to help you see everything against the backdrop of God.

Second, have an attitude of praise throughout the day. Before your feet hit the ground in the morning say, "Thank you, Lord, for this day and for letting me wake up and have another day to praise you on this earth."

Praise Him throughout the day for the little successes: being able to say no to those doughnuts on the counter, being able to feel full after just one small serving of your favorite dish, or being able to resist the urge to grab a snack on your way to bed.

Don't forget to praise Him!

Pause now for a moment in God's Word.

Daily Devotion — Day 33

Read Proverbs 3:1-8. Key Verses: Proverbs 3:5-6.

"Trust in the _____ with all your _____ and lean not on your own understanding; in all your ways _____ him, and he will make your _____ straight."

God never promised it would be easy; however, He did promise that His grace is sufficient for all. Grace is God's unmerited favor. It is God treating us better than we deserve. Jesus is saying to you today, "All you have to do is repent, my child, and ask me into your life, and I will carry your burdens." Our sinful nature separates us from God. Through grace it is as if we never sinned.

What are your obstacles to grace?

• Fear of failure

• Not wanting to give up old habits

• Fear of losing control, not wanting to totally surrender to God

Remember: Where sin is, God cannot be! Find victory in Jesus and overcome your obstacles of grace by praying without ceasing. Prayer is your perpetual line of open communication with God. Also, have an attitude of praise throughout the day; praise Him for the good and the bad.

Your spiritual challenge:
Pray for God to help you overcome your obstacles to grace today!

🍎 **Food Diary**	🙏 **Your Prayer**

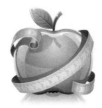

Day 34

Find Your Real Joy!

In 1 Thessalonians 5:16-18, Paul tells us:

Be joyful always; pray continually; give thanks in all circumstances, for this is God's will for you in Christ Jesus.

Do you hear what Paul is telling us? Scripture is telling us to be joyful always and to praise God in all circumstances!

The following is a story about a couple searching for joy and happiness. See if you can relate to this story about a young married couple.

Happily Ever After

She was eighteen years old, he was barely twenty on their wedding day. They went into their marriage with two totally different mindsets. She was a good Christian girl, somewhat sheltered, seeing life through rose-colored glasses. She went into the marriage thinking how wonderful and happy they would be living in a little white house with a white picket fence, two dogs, one cat, and two children—a boy and girl, of course.

He, on the other hand, was not raised in the church. He had been on his own, having a good time at the local junior college for several years but was ready to settle down and find a wife who would make him happy and content. They were both determined to go to college, so they settled down in a small college town to live out this thing called "happily ever after."

Fast-forward seven years. By now they have moved back to their home town, the husband has been working for several years, the wife has finally received her master's degree, has a new job, a new baby, and a new house to keep clean. They are finally climbing the ladder of success, trying to secure all those things to make them "happy."

While still living in her glass house and with so many new obligations, the wife suddenly finds herself in a tailspin. The baby always wants her attention, the house takes forever to clean, and whoever invented the eight-to-five work day must not have been a woman with children.

With all the new responsibilities, the wife finds she has very little time for her husband or to nourish the marriage. The husband, still searching for the happiness that is going to make him content, feels neglected, unloved, and starts spending more time at the office, the deer camp, and the golf course than at home with his new family.

They start going down a road that leads them further and further away from their marriage until the inevitable happens: their glass house shatters and the marriage is headed for the big Ds: divorce and disaster.

It's over. Their happiness is swept away in a few short months. The rose-colored glasses can no longer hide the pain and heartache. It is over, final, finished, that's it. No joy, no happiness to be found.

But is it really over? What about the commitment, the "happily ever after"? God begins to plant seeds of doubt in the husband, prompting him to come back, asking the wife to give this thing called marriage one more chance. In a last-ditch effort to save the marriage, they go to counseling with their pastor and are able to bring healing to the marriage.

The divorce is eventually canceled. Life begins once again as husband and wife have a new commitment—a deeper, stronger relationship and a new, more genuine "happily ever after." Each trial God allowed this couple to face was used to draw them closer to Him.

It took another eleven years for the husband to realize the hole he had been trying to fill all these years could only be filled by his Lord and Savior. Oh, what a joyous day it was when the husband came back to Christ. Only then was he able to find the true joy and contentment he desired.

The wife learned many life lessons, the primary one being that when she truly submits to Christ, praising Him for every event and letting Him be Lord over every aspect of her life, only then will she find her true source of joy. This kind of joy gives a person strength to make it through trials and the glue that holds marriages and family together, keeping them pointed toward Christ. God has helped that couple find true, lasting joy in their marriage.

Like that couple, many of you are searching for happiness in all the wrong places. Maybe you think happiness will come from another person, material possessions, more activities, or even from the food you eat. That kind of happiness is temporary, and it can be taken away from you in the blink of an eye. Joy, unlike happiness, can never be taken from you. Joy will only grow stronger through your trials. In fact, it will carry you through the hard times. It will carry you through your journey of life.

I know because this author is the wife.

When you discover true joy in your life as I did, you will be able to praise God through all circumstances. You will discover praise releases God's power in your life! With God, nothing is impossible! Therefore, don't get discouraged or overwhelmed. Set small, achievable goals. For example, I am striving to lose one pound this week.

Once you reach that goal, give God the glory and praise. Celebrate your success. After reaching several small goals, reward yourself with a new shirt, book, or something special instead of food. Take it one day at a time.

Jesus says in Matthew 6:34,

Therefore do not worry about tomorrow, for tomorrow will worry about itself. Each day has enough trouble of its own.

Having an active, healthy lifestyle is a choice you must make every day.

RECIPE CORNER
Oriental Slaw

6 cups slaw mix
green onions, chopped
½ cup sunflower seeds or walnuts
½ cup almonds

In a jar mix:
½ cup olive oil
3 tbsp. vinegar
½ tsp. salt (if desired)
½ tsp. pepper
2 tbsp. Splenda or Equal
1 seasoning packet from a package of chicken ramen noodles
(set noodles aside for later)

In a large bowl mix all ingredients together except for the noodles. Just prior to serving, crumble the ramen noodles over slaw mixture and toss.

Pause now for a moment in God's Word.

Daily Devotion — Day 34

Read Philippians 1:6 and fill in the blanks.

"Being _____ of this, that he who began a _____
_____ in you will carry it on to _____ until the day of
Christ Jesus."

Read what Paul writes in Philippians 3:12-14 and fill in the blanks.

"Not that I have already obtained all this, or have already been
made _____, but I _____ on to take hold of that for
which _____ _____ took hold of me. Brothers, I do
not consider myself yet to have taken hold of it. But one thing I
do: _____ what is _____ and _____
toward what is ahead, I press on toward the goal to _____
the _____ for which God has called me _____
in Christ Jesus."

You may never be exactly where you want to be in your battle with your
weight because your completion of the race will be in God's timing, not in
yours. But you can press on and persevere, keeping your eyes on Christ and
being confident He who has begun a good work in you will carry it out to
completion.

Your nutrition challenge:
Eat at least two servings of fruit every day this week.

171

🍎 **Food Diary**	🙏 **Your Prayer**

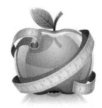

Day 35

The End—or the Beginning?

Have you ever been mountain climbing? Compare your journey toward weight lose and a healthy lifestyle to mountain climbing.

If you were a mountain climber climbing your mountain toward weight management, where would you describe yourself on the rope ascending the mountain? Are you the person dangling on the end of the rope saying, "I've been working on having a healthier lifestyle, have even made some significant changes, but have not lost a pound. I just can't do it. I'm tired, I'm frustrated, and I'm ready to quit."

Or are you a knot or two up on the rope? You've started making progress, you've seen you can do it, you have a long way to go, but you will press on.

Or are you the person near the top of the rope? You are making great strides; you've almost reached your goal and you feel great.

Do you know what a belayer is? The belayer is an essential part of the climbing team, the person who keeps the climber safely on a wall or rock face by holding a safety line. The belayer is connected to an anchor. As the climber ascends, the belayer pays out or takes in rope ready to apply a stopping force to the rope in case the climber falls. A belayer demands constant vigilance for the safety of the climber.

God is your belayer. Christ is with you wherever you are on the rope. Isn't it awesome to know He is always there, watching over you, encouraging you, and ready to step in if He needs to? With God holding the rope, you're guaranteed success up your mountain—to your goal—no manner how high or steep it is.

If you are at the bottom of this rope just barely hanging on, then God is underneath you, standing on the ground, pushing you up and there to catch you if you fall. If you're in the middle, He may be sending an angel to cheer you on, to encourage you along the way. The angel may be in the form of a friend who comes along at just the right time to encourage you or distract you. Angels may be in the form of a coworker or a spouse. It may be the comfort and peace you feel within you that encourages you along the way. Team up with God as you climb your mountain.

Pause now for a moment in God's Word.

Daily Devotion — Day 35

Read Philippians 4:10-13. Key Verse: Philippians 4:13.

Fill in the blanks:

I can do _____ through him who gives me _____.

With Christ, ANYTHING is possible!

Do you sometimes feel your prayers are not making it all the way to heaven? You pray and pray without an obvious answer. If God has not answered your prayers, ask Him, "God, how are you going to use this for your glory? How can I be used to glorify You through this?"

Sometimes God delays answers to your prayers to increase your faith. Sometimes God doesn't answer right away because He wants you to see Him. If God has not answered your prayer, trust it is for a reason; ask God to show you His glory. Never underestimate the power of praise and prayer in your life.

When you pray, ask for God's intervention into a situation, and praise Him for His power to work in every situation in your life for His glory. His power will be released into your life in whole new way. You will be amazed. Your job is to believe in His power. It is your lack of faith that sometimes inhibits God's work in your life. Discover the power in praise today!

Your nutrition challenge:
Don't eat any sweets today.

Food Diary	Your Prayer

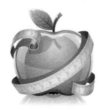

DAY 36

Pressing On Toward Your Goal

Look up Numbers 11:11-25, Key Verse: Numbers 11:23

The Lord answered Moses, "Is the Lord's arm too short? You will now see whether or not what I say will come true for you."

Do you feel overwhelmed, defeated, and ready to give up? If you are trying to conquer life alone, you are setting yourself up for failure. However, if you invite God along, He will fight your battles for you. God's arms are long enough to reach around any problem you may have.

As you continue on your journey toward weight loss you will want to do the following:

- Forget the past. Focus on the future.
- Enjoy where you are at each stage of your journey.
- Don't sweat the small stuff.
- Don't focus on how far you have to go to reach your goal. Focus on getting to the next knot. Take it one day at a time, hour by hour, minute by minute. Work on achieving one small goal at a time. Focus on being heaven bound since your ultimate reward will be in heaven.
- Always put God first in your life.
- Set realistic goals.

Remember, getting control of your weight problem is not something that is going to happen overnight. It is going to take a minute by minute, hour by hour, day by day commitment.

Pause now for a moment in God's Word.

Daily Devotion — Day 36

Read Psalm 33:1-11. Key Verse: Psalm 33:1.

Sing joyfully to the Lord, you righteous; it is fitting for the upright to praise Him.

Can you feel an overflowing of joy in your life? Joy is certainly something you are meant to feel. It is to be a happy, overflowing, pleasant experience. But joy does not depend on feelings. You are not to rejoice because you feel joyful. You can expect to eventually feel joyful as a result of your rejoicing. Joy is triggered by your life of praise.

The secret of true joy is not to do what you like to do, but to learn to like what you have to do. Happiness is not an end in itself; it is a by-product of something far greater. The real secret to happiness is to "seek first the kingdom of God." How do we do this? Submit yourself without reserve to Jesus Christ as King of your life every day. This will lead to joy, the path to true happiness. That joy will allow you to bloom where you are planted, with the circumstances you find yourself in, and regardless of your surroundings.

Receive the love, peace, and joy Jesus is offering you. Believe Jesus is with you, and God is working in every circumstance of your life to meet your needs. The very thing you think is painful proof of God's absence from your life is in fact His loving provision to draw you toward Himself, so your joy may be full. Look up and praise Him so His power can be released in your life through your praises. He loves you, and He dwells in the praises of His people.

Your spiritual challenge:
Ask God to help you
bloom where you are planted today.

Your nutrition challenge:
Encourage your friends and family to eat healthy food.

🍎 Food Diary	🙏 Your Prayer

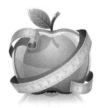

DAY 37

Set Small, Achievable Goals

Don't set yourself up for failure by setting unrealistic, impossible goals which are unrealistic and impossible to reach, such as losing ten pounds per week. Set small, reachable goals. For example, if you do not exercise, you might want to set a goal to start exercising fifteen minutes per day. Most everyone can find fifteen minutes of extra time in their day to exercise. Try it for a couple of weeks, and increase your time to twenty minutes per day and so on. All it takes is committing to one small change at a time to get you on the road to success.

Step by step, day by day, you can gradually implement new, healthy habits to last a lifetime. Making one change may help you lose a little for a short period of time, but it is the accumulation of several lifestyle changes that are going to really help you to lose weight and keep it off for a lifetime.

Let's look at some other small goals you might want to set:

- Drink at least eight cups of water every day.
- Eat at least one piece of fruit every day.
- Eat at least two colored vegetables every day.
- Take your lunch to work with you two to three days a week.
- Drink at least one cup of low fat or skim milk each day.
- Switch from sweet tea to unsweetened tea.
- Eat three small meals every day.
- Cut out at least one snack per day.

The devil wants you to be totally focused inward on your own desires, causing you to put food at the center of your life. He will tempt you with food every time you turn around and cause you to crave it. When you eat something good, he is going to tell you, "Oh, that was so good, have another piece. It won't hurt you, just this once."

How do you combat that? By saying, "Oh, that was so good. I think I will fix a piece to have tomorrow for lunch."

Look up Matthew 6:25 and fill in the blanks. Jesus said,

"Therefore I tell you, do not _____ about your _____, what you will eat or drink; or about your body, what you will wear. Is not _____ more important than food, and the _____ more important than clothes?"

Change your focus from inward to upward.

Look up Philippians 1:6 and fill in the blanks.

". . . being _____ of this, that he who began a good work in you will carry it on to _____ until the day of Christ Jesus."

Because your completion of this journey will be on God's time not in yours, you may never be exactly where you want to be in your battle with your weight. But you can persevere and keep your eyes on Christ.

Daily Devotion — Day 37

Read 1 Corinthians 10:31-11:1. Key Verse: 1 Corinthians 10:31.

So whether you _____ or _____ or whatever you do, do it all for the glory of God.

The choices you make today have the ability to greatly impact your future. Maintaining a healthy weight is one of the keys to prevention and control of many diseases.

Set Small, Achievable Goals

Your spiritual challenge:
Ask God what commitment He wants you to make today.

Your fitness challenge:
Push yourself to get up and get moving today.
You can't be active sitting down!

Eat today for a healthier tomorrow. Honor God with your food.

Food Diary	Your Prayer

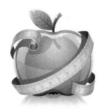

Day 38

Facts That Are Good To Know

Below is a quick review of some of the facts you should have learned on your journey to a healthier weight.

1. How many calories per gram do you get from:

- Carbohydrates   4 calories/gram
- Protein?   4 calories/gram
- Fat?   9 calories/gram

2. What percent of carbohydrates, proteins and fats should you have in your diet daily?

- Carbohydrates   55%
- Protein   20%
- Fat   25%

3. How many grams would that be for a 1,800 calorie diet?

- 1,800 x Carbohydrate (55%) =   990 ÷ 4 = 248 grams
- 1,800 x Protein (20%) =   360 ÷ 4 = 90 grams
- 1,800 x Fat (25%) =   450 ÷ 9 = 50 grams

4. Approximately how many grams of carbohydrates are in one serving of bread? 15 grams

5. How many calories in one pound? 3,500 Therefore, you must decrease your calories by 500 calories a day to lose one pound per week.

The more you know about the food you eat, the better you will be at controlling your diet. Your journey to diet freedom has begun with this book. Because this is a lifestyle and not just a diet, to be successful, your journey must continue for the rest of your life.

Daily Devotion — Day 38

Read Psalm 37:23-34. Key Verses: Psalm 37:23-24.

If the Lord delights in a man's way, He makes his _____ firm; though he stumbles, he will not _____ for the Lord upholds him with His hand.

Have you invited God to be a part of your journey to a healthier weight? Are you letting Him direct your path, so He will be there for you when you stumble and keep you from falling? Commit yourself to God today; let Him keep you on your continued journey to wellness.

Your spiritual challenge:
Invite God to be a vital part of your
every day journey to a better weight.

Your fitness challenge:
If you are having problems exercising due to the weather;
find a channel on your TV that offers exercise classes
or an exercise DVD that can be done
in your living room.

🍎 **Food Diary**	🙏 **Your Prayer**

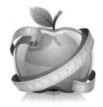

DAY 39

Daily Devotions Are Important

Look up Isaiah 43:18-19 and fill in the blanks.

Forget the _____ things [old habits]; do not _____ on the past. See, I am doing a new thing [God is doing a new thing in you]! Now it springs up; do you not perceive it? I am making a way in the desert [dry areas in your life] and _____ in the waste-land.

Daily devotions are an important part of your journey to a healthier weight. Once you have finished working through the forty days of devotions in this book, find another one or just began to read through your Bible. Let God's Word guide you as you continue on your journey. This journey cannot stop when the forty days are over. It has to continue throughout your life. Making daily devotion a part of your life will help enrich your life in numerous ways as you strive to draw closer to God.

Don't let your journey end with this book. Get active in your church. If you are not plugged into a church, you need to be. Pray about it, ask God to show you where He wants you to attend, and then be willing to step out in faith and start attending. Most churches offer small group Bible studies and/or daily devotional books to guide you through daily devotions for the rest of your life. Plant daily seeds of God's Word in your heart; these seeds will flourish and grow you into a new person who reflects Christ's image.

Daily devotion is important to help keep the dry areas of your life watered—at least it has been for me. Before I started daily devotions, I always felt illiterate when it came to the Bible because I didn't read it very much. I never realized how the Bible could be such a helpful tool and how when you get in tune with it, you are tuning into the heart of God. Before I started my spiritual journey, which prompted me to writing this program, I kept God just close enough to call on Him when I needed something. I didn't keep Him close enough so I could feel His presence just by breathing His name. I didn't really know Him.

But God started working on me though the trials, through daily devotions, and prayer journaling. God was able to get the "me" out of His way, so He could work through me.

You don't actually think I wrote this program and all those devotions myself do you? He did it, not me. When it is truly God prompting me to write something, the words will flow from me like magic. I know it has to be God, because I know I can't do it alone.

Through it all I have learned again and again when you step out in faith and do what God is prompting you to do, He will bless you. God wants to use you the same way. Show Him you can be faithful with the little things: with your diet and developing a healthy lifestyle. Let this be an opportunity for you to get in tune with God and be open for whatever He puts on your heart to do. Let Him use you to increase His kingdom and to bring Him glory. Bloom where you are planted, and let God use you to color His world.

Prayer journaling is also a very effective tool. Something about writing those prayers down makes them so much more powerful. It also helps you to track your prayers so that you will be more aware of those that have been answered. Take time to prayer journal so that you can see the power yourself.

Daily Devotion— Day 39

Read Joshua 24:15-27. Key Verse: Joshua 24:15.

"Choose for yourselves this day whom you will _____ . . . But as for me and my household we will serve the Lord."

If you are a Christian, you have made a choice to ask Jesus for forgiveness from your sins and come into your life to be your Lord and Savior. This relationship can change you into a new creation if you will permit it. Through Christ's work in your life you will discover gifts and talents you never knew existed. If you choose to put God at the center of your life, you will be amazed at what He can do with what you have to offer.

Step out in faith today, put your life in God's hands, and allow Him to work in a mighty way.

Your fitness challenge:
Increase your physical activity
by ten minutes every day this week.

Your spiritual challenge:
Make daily devotion and prayer
journaling a part of your life.

Food Diary	Your Prayer

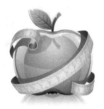

Day 40

Ask God for Help

But now, this is what the Lord says—he who created you, O Jacob, he who formed you, O Israel: "Fear not, for I have redeemed you; I have summoned you by name; you are mine. When you pass through the waters, I will be with you; and when you pass through the rivers, they will not sweep over you. When you walk through the fire, you will not be burned; the flames will not set you ablaze. For I am the Lord, your God, the Holy One of Israel, your Savior (Isaiah 43:1-3).

Have you asked God for help lately? Sometimes your prayer needs to be one word, "Help!"

Then they cried to the Lord in their trouble, and He saved them from their distress (Psalm 107:19).

God will not intervene in your life and help you unless you ask. He needs an invitation from you. Your journey to weight management must be a two-fold program to be successful. Unlike fad diets which rely on certain foods or gimmicks to help you lose weight, *The 40-Day Diet Makeover* is designed to help you develop a partnership with God so He can help you use the foods He has given you to glorify Him. However, until you humble yourself before Him and ask Him for help, He will not help you. He is waiting for an invitation from you. Speaking on prayer, Jesus said in Luke 11:10, "For everyone who asks receives."

Daily Devotion — Day 40

Read Matthew 4:1-4. Key Verse: Matthew 4:4.

Jesus answered, "It is written: 'Man does not live on bread alone, but on every word that comes from the mouth of God.'"

Don't center your life on food. Even Jesus was tempted with food by the devil. Strive today to avoid temptation and focus on God's ultimate plan for your life. Concentrate on seeking God's full will for your life. May everything you do glorify God!

Your spiritual challenge:
Pray God will help you change your focus from inward to upward as you continue on your personal journey toward a healthier weight.

So whether you eat or drink or whatever you do, do it all for the glory of God (1 Corinthians 10:31).

To God be the glory!

🍎 **Food Diary**	🙏 **Your Prayer**

REFERENCES

American Dietetic Association Nutrition Care Manual Web site. http/www.nutritioncaremaual.org/Diseases/CardiovascularDisease/Corona ryArteryDisease/Myocardial Infarction/Disease Process.

American Heart Association Web site. http://www.americanheart.org.

Arterburn, Stephen, and Pam Farrel, Devotions for Women on the Go. Tyndale House Publishers, Wheaton, IL, 2004.

Dietary Guidelines for Americans: Dietary Guidelines. http://www.mypyramid.gov.htm.

Marks-Katz, Marjorie, Fast Food Nutrition Guide. The Positive Line 79930, Item 1TP-27. http://www.thepositiveline.com.

Mississippi in Motion. Mississippi State University Extension Service, Riceland, 2005. http://msucares.com/health/health04/ms_in_motion/index.html

Pennington, Jean, Anna De Planter Bowes and Helen Nichols Church. Bowes & Church's Food Values of Portions Commonly Used. 16th ed. J.B. Lipponcott: Philadelphia, 1998.

Print Artist Gold. Sierra Home Version 12.0. by Sierra Entertainment, Copyright © Vivendi Universal Games, Inc. SA, 2002

United States Department of Agriculture Website: http://www.mypyramid.gov.

About the Author

PENNY W. DICKERSON grew up in church and accepted Jesus into her heart at the age of twelve. At times during her young life, she felt very close to God. Other times God was put on a shelf and only taken down when needed. He was not always the center of her life.

She married her husband, Kenny, right out of high school. Their first few years of marriage were spent in college. Penny, pursuing a career in nutrition, received her master's degree and became a registered dietitian. Kenny obtained his degree in accounting and became a CPA. After college, they settled down in a small town to begin a family. During the next ten years they were blessed with the birth of three sons--Spencer, Taylor, and Hunter.

Penny and her husband began their careers with the goal of achieving the American dream. However, they soon discovered something was missing in their pursuit of happiness. Church and God had not been priorities in their lives. Penny began to seek Jesus. She became more involved in the church and rekindled the fire, which had fizzled. God started working in her family's life and took them on an unexpected spiritual journey. After eighteen years of marriage, God raised her husband to be the spiritual leader of the household as He worked in both their lives in a mighty way.

Over the course of time, Penny felt that God wanted her to combine her twenty years experience in the field of nutrition and knowledge of His Word to help His people who struggle with their weight. Penny loves God and has a heart for God's people who struggle with weight issues. She wants to empower others through this study and daily devotions.

To contact the author, visit her website:
www.pennydickerson.com

Notes

Notes